NURSES IN BUSINESS

Edited by

Margo C. Neal, RN, MN

NURSECO, Inc.

Pacific Palisades, CA

First printing June 1982
Second printing August 1982

Printed in the United States of America

NURSECO, Inc.
PO Box 145
Pacific Palisades, CA 90272

Library of Congress Cataloging in Publication Data
Main entry under title:

Nurses in business.

  Bibliography: p.
  Contents: The socialization of nurses / Margo C. Neal — Health Communicators Foundation Inc. / Donna M. Tarulli — Joint practice with a physician / Shirley St. Amand — [etc.]
    1. Nursing—Practice.   2. Nursing—Practice—United States.   3. Nursing—Economic aspects—United States.   I. Neal, Margo Creighton, 1935—
RT86.7.N87   610.73'068   81-16954
ISBN 0-935236-21-X (pbk.)   AACR2

To
those nurses who want
the freedom of independence
and who are willing
to take the risks involved;
and in memory of
Shirley St. Amand
whose innovative leadership and pioneering
in the nursing profession
were cut short by her untimely death
during the production of this book.

Nursing Resource Books from Nurseco:

Nursing Care Planning Guides, Set 1 *2nd Edition*   0-935236-09-0
Nursing Care Planning Guides, Set 2 *2nd Edition*   0-935236-16-3
Nursing Care Planning Guides, Set 3   0-935236-05-8
Nursing Care Planning Guides, Set 4   0-935236-07-4
Nursing Care Planning Guides, Set 5   0-935236-14-7

and the following specialty editions extrapolated from the above:
Nursing Care Planning Guides for Long-Term Care   0-935236-13-9
Nursing Care Planning Guides for Psychiatric
   and Mental Health Care   0-935236-15-5
Nursing Care Planning Guides for Medical-Surgical Care   0-935236-23-6
Nursing Care Planning Guides for Maternity and Pediatrics Care 0-935236-24-4

Memory Bank for Critical Care   *2nd Edition*   0-935236-22-8
Memory Bank for Hemodynamic Monitoring   0-935236-20-1
Memory Bank for HemoDialysis   0-935236-18-8

Nurses in Business   0-935236-21-X
Perspectives on Continuing Education in Nursing   0-935236-12-0

Contents

Part B   Foundations for Establishing Your Own Business

Contributing Authors

Patricia A. Allen, RN, MS. *Partner, Perinatal Dimensions, Philadelphia, PA.*

Julie Bornstein, BA, MA, JD. *Partner, Bornstein & Gurewitz, Attorneys at Law, Los Angeles, CA.*

Rona Lee Cohen, RN, MN, FPNP. *Director, Seminars on Sexuality, Beverly Hills, CA.*

Sharon Goldsmith, RN, MS. *Founder-Director, Seminars on Sexuality, Beverly Hills, CA.*

Arleen Gordon, RN, MPH. *Consultant, San Francisco, California.*

Margo C. Neal, RN, MN. *Founder and President, Nurseco, Inc., Pacific Palisades, CA.*

Frank E. Norton, PhD. *Associate Professor, Graduate School of Management, University of California, Los Angeles, CA.*

Joan Reighley, RN, MN. *Psychotherapist and Nurse Educator, Private Practice, Los Angeles, CA.*

Christopher M. Smith, MBA. *Vice-President, National Nursing Review, Inc., Los Altos, CA.*

Sandra F. Smith, RN, MS. *President, National Nursing Review, Inc., Los Altos, CA.*

Shirley St. Amand, RN, MN. *Cardiology Nurse Practitioner, Private Practice, Los Angeles, CA.*

Donna M. Tarulli, RN, MN. *President and Educational Director, Health Communicators Foundation, Inc., Los Angeles, CA.*

Katharine Borges Thompson, RN, MN, MFCC. *Clinical Nurse Specialist, Private Practice, Marina del Rey, CA.*

Dorothy B. Turner, RN, MS. *Partner, Perinatal Dimensions, Philadelphia, PA.*

Mary-Scott Welch, AB. *Free-lance writer; author of NETWORKING: THE GREAT NEW WAY FOR WOMEN TO GET AHEAD (Harcourt Brace Jovanovich, 1980; Warner Books, 1981).*

Foreword

I was both honored and excited to be given the opportunity to write a foreword for this unique and timely book. That such a book is relevant and marketable to nurses is, in itself, a landmark. Ten years, even five years ago, such a publication would have been impossible. Nurses were not in business, and more important, thought business values incompatible with the values of a profession. Fortunately, both behavior and values have changed.

According to recent statistics, 95% of all businesses in the United States are considered small (less than $125,000.00 in capital). The number of small business ventures has increased enormously over the past few years. The risk of small business failure, however, is very high, with only one out of every six businesses surviving more than five years. But, the potential rewards are also great. Not only is there possibility of financial success, but there is independence and the satisfaction of doing what you like doing.

There is no magic formula for business success. It takes a lot of hard work, good luck, adequate financing, and a great deal of self-confidence. The successful entrepreneur asks what is now being done or provided that is desirable, timely, and needed — then goes out and does it or provides it.

Being in business isn't for everyone, but it is another option to consider. For nurses who care about both people and profits, having your own business may be the answer to "what should I be when I grow up?" If the idea of being in business intrigues and excites you, this book will be of great value. As a nurse you already acquired skills in working with people. These skills are a tremendous asset that combined with venture capital, a willingness to take a chance, and the excellent advice given in this text will help make your business venture a success.

Each author in this book shares a wealth of meaningful wisdom and experience. Use this book to identify the gaps in required business knowledge and skill. Fill in the gaps and give it a try. Whatever the ultimate outcome you will have added an exciting new dimension to your life.

Dorothy J. del Bueno, EdD, RN
Editor of *A Financial Guide*
for Nurses: Investing In
Yourself and Others

Preface

The number of nurses in business is growing. Yet, relatively little has been written about them. Nor is there much available for nurses who wish to explore this option. In essence, the phenomenon of a nurse being in an independent business *in nursing* is so new that very little literature on the subject exists.

The main purpose of this book is to provide encouragement, motivation, and role modeling for nurses who are exploring this new option. Other purposes are to look at some of the forces that affected nurses and their orientation to business and to present some how-tos that can help them make the transition to business, should they choose.

Although the number of nurses in business today is growing, there is little known about them and how they got to their present positions. What were the motivating forces? How did they overcome the obstacles? How did they make the transition? What are the socializing forces that helped or hindered? While this book is not the result of any research study, it does provide some interesting answers to these and other questions from a group of nurse-entrepreneurs.

These interesting portraits of nurses-turned-businesspersons recall some of the circumstances that propelled them to their present positions. There are differences and similarities. One of the most interesting of the latter is that the majority of these nurses were not prepared to enter a business; they came to it by roundabout means and frequently because of unsatisfactory professional work environments elsewhere.

That is often the way new careers emerge and become a permanent part of the landscape. I think we can safely say that this option for nurses is here to stay and that more and more nurses will prepare for an independent business practice while still students.

During the eleven years since I started my business, I have answered many questions that could have been answered with this book, and I have encouraged nurses to try the independent route; I've told them they can do it. So I suppose the most compelling reasons for putting this book together is to show that yes, nurses can function independently, and be successful in the endeavor. I wanted to show, too, that there is a variety of nursing businesses that are available, dependent to a great degree on one's imagination, energy, and creativity. My hope is that this book will say, "It is possible."

I wish to acknowledge each of the contributing authors to this book. Each one has spent many hours on the preparation of their respective chapters, and happily undertook the task in the midst of busy schedules.

Margo C. Neal

Part A

**Traditional Socialization
and
Current Nontraditional Practices**

1

The Socialization of Nurses

Margo C. Neal

Sugar and spice, and everything nice.
That's what little girls are made of.

And little girls become nurses, and nurses, too, traditionally were grown-up versions of "sugar and spice, and everything nice." Nurses have also been described in other traditional female terms, such as *dependent, sensitive, empathic, passive, subjective, emotional, non-aggressive, noncompetitive, submissive.* These traditional traits translated into "human compassion." "Good" nurses became socialized by institutions to be selfless workers who were always willing to sacrifice their own needs for the sake of the patient. "Good" nurses were not concerned with salaries, working conditions, weekends off.[1]

The Socialization Process

How did nurses get this way? Many forces have been at work, for a long time.

In the Beginning

The process of socialization [is] the development of an individual from child to adult in a certain culture whose values selectively emphasize certain things and whose rules and procedures have been established in order to attain them.   [Hennig and Jardim 1977]

[1] Although nursing is no longer the exclusive domain of women, men still make up a very small percentage of its ranks. And so what follows is primarily about female nurses.

3

Socialization involves values, beliefs, attitudes, and behaviors. In our society, females have been socialized to be passive, unassuming, quiescent, submissive, and nonassertive, and these qualities have come to be labeled "feminine." Males, on the other hand, have been encouraged and rewarded for being just the opposite—assertive, aggressive, active, questioning, and competitive—and these qualities are accepted as "masculine."

Social forces in our environment help prepare us for future roles. Betty Harragan (1977) points out that little boys are socialized from early on to participate in the corporate world. For example, traditionally they are members of sports teams and are taught competitive play. Competitive, that is, toward the opposing team but not toward their own team members. They are taught that the team is everything, that even if they do not like the people on their team, they need them to play the game, to get the job done, to win. Winning, teamwork, playing to win—these are attributes that society today places on men, and on business.

What are little girls taught? They are taught to be caring, to be full of human compassion, to be selfless. Much of this philosophy is rooted in the Judeo-Christian ethic that is pervasive in our society. For the most part, little girls have not participated in team sports. They have played in one-to-one sports where the emphasis is not on winning but on *how well* they play the game. They have been taught that competitive and team sports are for boys, that it is unfeminine to participate in such events. (Since females in our society have not been socialized to function effectively within a team, it is not difficult to understand why the concept of team nursing encountered such great difficulty in implementation.) Girls have been taught one element of competition, though—to compete with other little girls for the attention of little boys.

These same little girls have been socialized into appropriate female roles, for example, playing nurse; if a little boy participated, he was expected to play the doctor.

Traditionally, career options for these little girls have been limited to secretarial work, teaching, or nursing. Unlike boys, who have been socialized to have a responsible career and support their families, girls have been taught that they needed a career only to support themselves until they could marry and be supported. Many were taught and encouraged to have the skills of a nurse "in case something happened to their husbands." In other words, only as an insurance policy, the case of last resorts.

In Nursing School

The majority of the nurses in the United States and Canada today are products of hospital training schools. The emphasis in these schools was clinical expertise in a prescribed manner, some theoretical components, minimum creative problem solving, and deference to the physician. (Do you remember standing up when a doctor walked in?) These nurses were trained to varying degrees to be the "handmaiden of the physician," a term much discussed and debated in later years. The graduates of these schools were socialized to work in hospitals or in doctors' offices. In fact, many of them got married and worked very little or not at all.

As nursing schools began to move away from "training" nurses in hospitals to "educating" them in the mainstream of higher education, new dimensions were added to the curricula. For example, the students were taught the scientific method of problem solving and to apply this method to patient care. They were taught the difference between dependent and independent nursing functions; moreover, they were taught to make independent nursing judgments and to carry them out without a doctor's order. They were taught to spell out the rationale for their decisions. In essence, they were taught to think, to have options, and to implement and evaluate their subsequent nursing actions. Less emphasis was placed on clinical expertise with its multiple hours of practice required for such high competence, and more emphasis was placed on scientific problem solving. This new way of perceiving a patient became refined and students were subsequently taught to view the patient from a particular theoretical framework and to carry out the nursing process within that frame of reference. And still they were socialized to work in hospitals.

All of this took time, of course, and some of that time was taken from that previously allotted to clinical hours in the training schools. This wrought great conflict in the reality of the workaday world of the acute care hospital.

On the Units

The battle lines were drawn between the nurses who had clinical expertise and little theory, chiefly products of the diploma programs, and the nurses who were long on theory but shorter on clinical expertise. The battle still rages today, attenuated periodically and temporarily by such issues as strikes, continuing education, and supplemental staffing agencies.

The new graduate has a difficult time adjusting to the "reality shock" (Kramer 1974) of life in a general hospital. She is expected to function almost immediately in a way that is quiet, unquestioning, nonassertive, obedient, submissive. Many times the greatest amount of pressure to perform in this manner is exerted by her peers: "We've always done it this way." "We've been doing it this way for years." The traditional socialization forces are alive and well. Or are they all that alive and well?

The Change Over

Nothing much occurred to change the profile of the typical, traditional nurse until the late 1960s. That's when nurses first went on strike, initially in New York, later in San Francisco. It was the economic revolution in nursing, and it sent shock waves through both the professional and lay communities.

Gradually these groups of nurses began to be looked on as heroines of their profession. They gained respect, and the germ of a radical idea — radical to nurses, that is — began to take shape: "Yes, it is OK for nurses to be concerned about money." But everyone knows that nurses don't care about money, that they only care about patients! Change! Radical idea! Unheard of! Nurses began to raise their consciousness in the sphere of economic realities.

The sixties breakthrough carried over to the seventies. Nurses demanded and received more pay. They received more education. With the latter they wanted more autonomy, since their education taught them to think independently, to be creative problem solvers, to make independent judgments. They were educated and socialized to be leaders in nursing, to set new standards of care, to provide primary care to patients, care based on scientific rationale and mixed with psychosocial aspects that would make the patient and the public feel that "good old-fashioned nurses" were back. It was the era of producing the clinical specialist. And the clinical specialist, like the majority of nurses even today, was socialized to work for hospitals, or other health-related agencies, or for doctors. The implication was that nurses always have, do, and always will work for someone else.

Forces of Change

About this same time, social forces were at work to change the status of women. These forces worked concurrently to change the status of men, too, as roles were examined, redefined, modified, and changed.

The women's liberation movement affected nearly all members of society, whether they supported it or not.

The *Virginia Slims American Women's Opinion Poll* (1980) revealed some profound changes in women in general in the decade between 1970 and 1980:

- *Example:* In 1970, it was the younger, more-educated women who were in favor of changing women's status. By 1980, older, less-educated women supported the change in greater numbers than the younger group.

- *Example:* The 1980 woman "...has become increasingly sensitive to being treated as an inferior."

- *Example:* The 1980 woman has become aware of the cultural mores that have defined her role in society. She believes that traditional socialization patterns, rather than inherent sex characteristics, have shaped the stereotypical male and female patterns of behavior.

- *Example:* In 1980, "...women have been altering social attitudes by redefining traditional perceptions of what have generally been considered to be male and female domains."

- *Example:* Increasing numbers of women are entering the traditional male domains of business, finance, and government, and this trend is expected to continue.

The processes of change (Toffler 1970) and their directions (Toffler 1980) have greatly influenced our society in general. According to Toffler's view, people want a piece of the "power" pie; they no longer want to be homogeneous. He sees the demands of groups for recognition, for expanded roles and responsibilities as an effort to gain some power — power that will permit those involved to have greater control over their own destinies, over their own lives, than was previously available.

This effort to gain power can be seen in many levels of the nursing profession. As nurses enter new roles within the profession, they want to have the corresponding power. They want to work on a collegial level with other members of the health team, not in a subordinate role. Even those who do not function in some of the expanded and new roles are "getting into the power act." For example, one could review the tremendous shift of nurses to working for supplementary staffing agencies, rather than directly for hospitals, as a way to gain more personal power and control over their professional lives.

Change creates new roles. In the nursing profession there are now countless roles that were nonexistent ten, fifteen, twenty years ago: roles such as patient advocate, nurse practitioner, clinical specialist, continuing education specialist, patient educator, psychotherapist. Within the job description of a staff nurse in acute care general hospitals are functions that have gradually been taken over from the physicians — IVs, defibrillation, insertion of nasogastric tubes, to name a few.

Change permeated the content that was taught in nursing schools, too. Students were prepared for new roles such as nurse practitioner and with it the possibility of setting up an independent practice. However, "few nurse practitioners have chosen to set up private practices, possibly because they have little opportunity to learn management and business skills in their education programs" (Simms 1977, p. 114). Thus, although nurses acquired the knowledge and skills to function independently, they lacked the essential non-nursing skills of business. They continued, for the most part, to work in clinics, to work for others.

Simms did a study to find out whether any nursing schools provided business management courses for their students, and whether faculty and students did in fact desire such courses. She found that there was then no minor in business for a nursing student, and that nursing students who chose business or management classes as electives might find that they would not be credited toward their degree. In addition, "The overall conclusions would seem to be that both students and faculties in nursing programs prefer more courses that would help nurses to become entrepreneurs in the practice of nursing" (Simms 1977, p. 118). It makes sense. If nurse practitioners are to have a significant impact on the public, they need to function in innovative environments, to move out of traditional work places. But survival in an independent practice in a business setting often depends heavily on having some business knowledge and skills.

Not everyone within the profession agrees with the new roles, with the changes. At a national nursing convention in Minneapolis in 1973, a California nursing educator deplored the exodus of master's-prepared nurses from the hospital. At that time, most of these nurses were leaving to work for other agencies; few were going to set up their own businesses. However, the exodus continued and now appears to be firmly entrenched in the nursing landscape.

In all fairness, it must be said that many hospitals have made innovative changes to accommodate the nurse who wants to problem solve, to create new ways of providing patient care. And these changes satisfied many. Others felt the need to become completely independent, to function on their own, to be nurse-entrepreneurs. They felt the environment was still reinforcing the old ways; that is, it was reinforcing them to be accepting, unquestioning, and submissive, and would allow them to be innovative and creative within a too-narrow scope. When asked about the prime motivators that led her to start her own business, one young, bright, well-educated (master's level) nurse replied, "In the hospitals where I worked, I wasn't permitted to function the way I had been prepared and wanted to do."

Flying the Coop

By the late 1970s, there was much evidence that something new and different was occurring in the profession. And that something was the fact that many nurses were becoming self-employed. Not only as private-duty nurses, but as entrepreneurs, as private practitioners, as businesspeople.

They were independent of the hospital system of which they had been a part for so long. They had flown the coop. "The early independent nursing practices were primarily clinical in nature, notably psychiatric and medical/surgical but a few independent practices in the area of inservice education also surfaced" (Neal 1981).

The climate was changing for nurses. Although some early nurse-entrepreneurs were looked on with suspicion, as the decade of the eighties approached it became almost *trendy* to be in business for yourself. Variations on any of these themes could (and still can) be heard over and over again:

- "I'm running this (CE) division but I don't get to share the profits."
- "I can do the same thing for myself."
- "I've opened three staffing offices for corporations, and I'm not doing it again unless it's for my own business."
- "There must be something else I can do."
- "I'd like to be in business for myself."
- "I'd like to set up an independent practice."
- "I'm tired of being subordinate."
- "If she can do it, why can't I?"
- "I'd like to free lance."

The early nurse-entrepreneurs were willing to take the risks of "going independent." Instead of viewing risk from the traditional negative, female perspective of a loss, damage, injury, or hurt, as something to be avoided (Hennig and Jardim 1977), they began to incorporate risk into their lives from the male perspective — that is, as a danger *or* opportunity, as a potential loss *or* gain — as a result of judgment based on past dealings with risk rather than as a forgone conclusion of personal loss.

By the mid-1970s, a few articles could be found in the nursing literature relating to independent practices. In the late 1970s, nursing conventions began to include such content in their programs. And in the 1980s, we can even read articles about starting your own business that are geared specifically to nurses (Neal 1981). It is interesting how quickly the climate can change! Take the hotly debated issue of supplementary staffing agencies. At first, they were denigrated by hospitals and nursing organizations, by most people in fact, except the nurses who worked for them. And today, some nursing leaders are saying, "How many of them are owned by nurses?" It is a measure of how far nursing has changed in its widening orientation that the question how many are *owned* by nurses, not simply *run* by nurses, can be asked.

Yes, Virginia, the nursing profession is changing and expanding and is open to innovation. Perhaps now, instead of losing nurses to social work, to real estate, to law, to the many other places they have gone, perhaps now the profession can accommodate them in roles and environments of their own choosing.

Nurse-Entrepreneurs

Several nurses have gone into business and gained visibility as en-trepreneurs. Are they special types of persons? Do they come from a particular background? Although no studies have been done to date on this specific group, the study of Hennig and Jardim (1977) sug-gests that at least the early nurse-entrepreneurs may have had something special or different in their backgrounds that led them toward their present businesses.

These authors studied intensely a group of twenty-five women who were in top corporate positions. The study found that the twenty-five had some major differences in their socialization com-pared to their female peers. For example, several of the women were treated "like sons" by their fathers (none of the women had brothers); that is, they were taught to view risk from the traditional male perspective, and to be competitive in sports. They were groomed to be leaders, not to be in a subordinate role. Their fathers became the primary role model in their lives. In school, college, and career, the women became leaders and developed many characteristics of a behavioral style that is usually reserved for men — that is, they were decisive, aggressive, innovative, and competitive.

They recalled the "special" relationship with their fathers, who took them on outings and excursions, who encouraged and rewarded them for being independent, and for exploring new vistas. This contrasted with their memories of their mothers whom they recalled in the traditional female model — that is, caring, protective, nonassertive, fearful of risk. In later life, these women did not feel that the traditional assumption of female inferiority applied to them.

The Entrepreneurial Pattern

"Studies of all kinds of business in diverse cultures reveal that people starting their own enterprises follow a common pattern" (Shapero 1980). This pattern is described in terms of four major factors: displacement, a strong propensity to take control of one's life, credibility, and resources.

Displacement follows many of life's situational crises — for example, divorce, death, loss of a job. There is a high incidence of entrepreneurship among refugees — people who have been displaced from their homeland. Other forms of displacement include being passed over for a job or a promotion, thus generating the *feeling* that it is time to "move on," "to look around." After experiencing a degree of displacement many people turn to some form of entrepreneurship. Often it takes some type of situational crisis to propel people out of the inertia of their daily lives into an entrepreneurial activity. How many times have you heard a variation of this theme? "Getting fired from that job was the best thing that ever happened to me?"

Taking control of one's life is a second characteristic of many entrepreneurs. These people see the locus of control as being internal rather than external, and they believe that they can control their own lives. They prefer to define their own parameters rather than have them defined by others.

More and more married nurses (as well as single parents in general) are continuing to work while raising children. They are beginning to view their work as a career, not merely as a job. A significant number are looking at the work they are doing, and asking themselves if this is what they want to be doing for the next fifteen, the next twenty, years. Many nurses are answering that they do not want to stay within their present bureaucratic system; they want to participate in a situation where they can make up the rules. They want more control over their professional lives.

Credibility is a belief that it is feasible to start and run a business. It involves being able to perceive yourself doing it, and it is often achieved in increments; that is, step by step as you achieve success and grow and build. It is often generated by role models or by mentors.

For nurses, the credibility pattern is just beginning to emerge. Although the largest segment of the public still thinks of nurses in the traditional role of hands-on caring for the sick, a smaller segment sees them as competent, independent health practitioners, evidenced by the increasing number of clients being treated by these practitioners. Nurses who are in business are staying there only because they are seen as credible by the consumers who buy their services.

Resources, chiefly financial ones, are essential. Sometimes the resources are acquired by "moonlighting," by credit, or by loans from family or friends. Whatever the source, they are essential; a certain amount of funding is needed to initiate any enterprise. Starting a business on the proverbial shoestring is becoming more and more difficult in today's inflationary times.

According to Shapero, scratch any entrepreneur and you'll find a significant amount of these four factors that make up the entrepreneurial pattern. Given that these characteristics are fundamental, there are other variables that help to shape the entrepreneur — variables such as socialization, family background, and education, along with role models and mentors.

As we've seen, nurses in general have not been socialized toward business, particularly toward entrepreneurship. Yet some have gone in this direction and more and more will follow. What can these nurses do to help themselves become independent businesspersons?

Bridging the Gap

How do nurses make the transition from employee to self-employed, or even employer? There are numerous ways.

For one, they join **networks** (discussed in chapter 11).

Role modeling is another way. There are still very few nurse-entrepreneurs who can serve as role models to aspiring ones. It's probably necessary to role model some facets of several people you know. A great motivator is, "If she can do it, I can do it."

Whom do you know, female or male, who is successful in business, in a corporation, in a small business, or in a private practice? How many nurses do you know who have admirable abilities that would be essential in setting up your own business, qualities such as decision-making ability, an ability to focus clearly on the problem at hand, the ability to work hard for long-term rewards versus short-term ones, the ability to take risks, the ability to work independently? Talk to these people; take them to lunch and ask them if they are willing to share some of their experiences with you. Role models can be inspiring, motivating, and validating.

Mentors can help. How? According to the dictionary a mentor is a wise and trusted counselor. A mentor takes you under her or his wing and guides you through the maze. If you can find a mentor, lucky you; it's not easy. Mentors are more apt to be found in corporations where contact between mentor and "mentee" is very frequent. A mentor can give guidance and advice, can tell you what pitfalls to avoid as well as what avenues to be sure to explore.

For nurses going into business, a mentor is not apt to be a nurse simply because, like role models, there just aren't that many around. One nurse who was an early entrepreneur related that her mentors were businessmen because not only did she not know any other nurses in business, she didn't know other women in business either.

Can you buy the services of a mentor? Yes, you can; management consultants can be viewed as paid mentors. You must, however, choose such a person with the same care that you use in choosing your accountant, your attorney, or any other professional adviser.

Professional business organizations are another way to become socialized to the new role of business person. Mentors and role models can sometimes be found in them. Nurses joining such groups may not find any other nurses there yet. But most important, they will find other people who can be invaluable contacts, resources, and referrals for them. They will find conversation not of staffing patterns, patient outcomes, or administrative guidelines, but about negotiating a contract, getting a loan, or developing a proposal. Such groups can help shape a nurse's thinking as she strives to learn more about business and about the formal and informal ways it operates.

For women, such groups can provide entry to an "old girl's

network," that is, to people who can provide you with those invaluable contacts, resources, and referrals. Although men have had such networking groups for years (Rotary and Kiwanis are two), there are no traditional groups for women. Within the last few years, however, many groups oriented to women in business have emerged, such as the Women in Business (WIB) in Los Angeles and AGOG (All the Good Old Girls) in Minneapolis.

Seminars, Institutes, Workshops, Courses. These groups can help nurses gain the business knowledge and skills that they never got in nursing school. They provide many of the basics needed to start out on your own. Many, many are available through universities, colleges, professional organizations, or the Small Business Administration (consult the Yellow Pages of the telephone directory for the latter). Or you can combine these routes with self-directed learning such as books. Many how-to books are available; an excellent one is *Introduction to Business* (Altfest and Lichner 1978). It is part of the Barnes and Noble Outline series and is widely available in bookstores across the country.

And in the Future

What can we expect regarding changes in the socialization of nurses for business? The trend that has started — changes in curriculum, new career options for nurses — can be expected to continue and expand.

It seems clear that more and more nurses will go into business, either as entrepreneurs or as part of the corporate world. Increasing numbers are being employed by large health care corporations and these nurses are requiring socialization to the corporate world and to both its formal and informal organizations.

A number of nurses are acquiring a master's in business administration (MBA). Just as this degree is opening up many new paths for women in general, so it is for nurses. An MBA can open up a new world to nurses planning either an entrepreneurial or a corporate career. A few schools are even now changing to allow nursing students to take a minor in business.

A small number of nurse-entrepreneurs are in their current positions because they planned early in their careers to be independent, to leave the traditional system. They are where they are because of careful planning and mapping to get there. But many others can recall their start in business as something they "fell into," as an "escape from the system," as "something that just happened," without planning. These nurses had to overcome great odds, and they join the others as role models.

We can expect that an increasing number of students, particularly at the graduate level, will opt for independent careers and will acquire course content that will be of significant help to them, such as basic accounting, financial forecasting and planning, marketing, and other business skills, as well as negotiation, and writing and presenting proposals. And how about a course in dreaming? Dreaming? Yes. Nurses and women have been socialized to live and work within a relatively narrow scope. Do they know that a great part of maintaining a business is literally dreaming up new ideas and translating them into concrete, marketable services or products?

A great boost can be expected for nurses with a clinical practice (nurse practitioners, psychotherapists) once third-party payment is available for nurses. Although a few insurance carriers do provide such reimbursement, it is still only a token effort. It is difficult for nurse practitioners, for example, to make the impact on health care that they are prepared to do, unless the client's insurance, Medicare, or its state counterpart, will cover it. The large numbers of poor people in the country, who stand to gain the most from such payment to nurses, are the ones who currently gain the least, for they cannot afford to pay for these services.

Other changes are coming for nurse-entrepreneurs, too. Currently, there is a bill before the legislature in at least one state (California) to permit nurses to incorporate, as physicians are able to do. Significantly, this bill was authored by a nurse who was elected to the state government.

So it appears that nurses are being socialized to some roles and behaviors that were formally the primary domain of men: decisive, assertive, leadership, independent, innovative roles—and they can still be caring, compassionate, and nurturing. Not all nurses are looking at their place in the profession merely as a time-limited "job;" rather, many are seeing it as a career that can coexist with marriage or children, or both.

Although nursing has been chiefly a profession for women, men are entering it in increasing numbers. Interestingly, as societal changes have evolved and relatively large numbers of women have entered medicine, there has not been a corresponding number of men entering nursing. Could this be related to the fact that there is a wide disparity in economic rewards between the two professions? If so, perhaps the advent of nurses into business will help even out the sexual makeup of medicine and nursing.

In the 1980s, nurses are on the move—politically, socially, career-option-wise. Nurses are thought of not only as caring, compassionate, and nurturing, but also as categories of characteristics are compatible: they are not mutually exclusive. New options are available and one of those, nurses in business, clearly is . . .

An idea whose time has come.

References

Altfest, Lewis J., and Lichner, Alan B. *Introduction to Business.* New York: Barnes & Noble, 1978.

Harragan, Betty L. *Games Mother Never Taught You.* New York: Warner Books, 1977.

Hennig, Margaret, and Jardim, Anne. *The Managerial Woman.* New York: Doubleday, 1977.

Kramer, Marlene. *Reality Shock.* St. Louis: Mosby, 1974.

Neal, Margo C. "Starting Your Own Business." In *A Financial Guide for Nurses,* Dorothy del Bueno, Ed. Boston: Blackwell, Scientific Publications, Inc. 1981

Shapero, Albert. "Have You Got What It Takes to Start Your Own Business?" *Savvy* 1, (4):33-37, April 1980.

Simms, Elsie. "Preparation for Independent Practice." *Nursing Outlook* 25, (2):114, 117-118, February 1977.

The 1980 Virginia Slims American Women's Opinion Poll; A Survey of Contemporary Attitudes. The Roper Organization, 1980.

Toffler, Alvin. *Future Shock.* New York: Random House, 1970.

Toffler, Alvin. *The Third Wave.* New York: William Morrow, 1980.

2

Health Communicators Foundation, Inc.

Donna M. Tarulli

At the onset, I never visualized how demanding starting a business would be. Now, in retrospect, after three years of developing HCFI—Health Communicators Foundation, Inc.—I truly believe that flexibility, strong commitment to an idea, and human support have enabled me to remain marginally sane throughout this project.

I have had the luxury of not having been alone in this endeavor: I have three partners who entered the project at different points in its development. Together, we have produced what we feel to be a viable business, which we based on some creative ideas we had about the health care system today. The excitement of creation is only exceeded by the thrill of the actual implementation of these ideas. It has been both our pleasure and our good fortune to see our business change, grow, and begin to prosper. That means that our long hours of hard work and the changes that we each had to make in our lives have begun to pay off. It also means that our ideas that nurses are and can continue to be instrumental in making creative changes in the health care industry are no longer assumptions, but reality.

The Impetus for Business

The impetus for this project grew out of some ideas that had been rolling around in my head for a while. I have always believed that nurses are, and always have been, the best health teachers around. Take their problem-solving ability, add their knowledge and their special way of dealing with people, and there's something there that's very marketable.

After a year and a half or so of working for gynecologic on-cologists, I found that many of my friends and colleagues would ask me for advice. I spent a lot of off-work time teaching consumers just how to get the most out of a visit to the doctor. In speaking with some of my friends, I found out they too were working overtime educating the public and were also sometimes called upon to share their valuable knowledge and skill with a hospital or industry in need of some special health-related information. I started thinking—in every other industry or profession, that is called a consultation and carries with it quite a nice fee for service. What happened to nurs-ing? Is it our fault for not demanding more for ourselves? So, the idea of marketing and selling what I had to offer was born. I found that as I shared this idea with friends, some were skeptical, some supportive, and some just thought I was crazy. Anyhow, I found a friend who shared my philosophy and together we continued to pur-sue ideas of a health consultation business.

Certainly nursing and business are philosophically and theoretical-ly worlds apart! How then does a successful marriage occur? A matchmaker, of course! Such a project takes two distinctly different bodies of knowledge and two different states of mind. I know where the nursing knowledge came from, but business, or what they call entrepreneurial activity, that is a mystery. Just what are the factors responsible for this entrepreneurial activity? After reading *The En-trepreneurial Woman,* by Sandra Winston, the mystery began to unravel.

Reams of research have been done in attempts to identify causes of motivation and entrepreneurial activity. A list of many complex and contradictory factors has been narrowed down to six by the most thoughtful observers in the field (Winston 1979). This list in-cludes role models, a willingness to take risks, feelings of indepen-dence, internal or external control, motivation, resources, and, lastly, something present in nursing today, feelings of displacement.

As I looked that list over and read Ms. Winston's book, I was able to understand just what may have caused me to pursue setting up a business. I seem to have had all the right ingredients to make the recipe work.

Role Models: Business

Fortunately, as a child, I was exposed to many role models; if entrepreneurship is inbred, then I certainly qualified. My first and best role model was my father. My father always owned his own business, was successful, and worked very hard. I realize now that I picked up much of my ability from him. He always displayed the ability to interact well with people, to negotiate, to delegate well, and always to remain fair and honest in business transactions. He displayed amazing concern for his fellowman. It was through my father's fine example that my brother and I were able to learn skills that can never be taught in school.

I grew up hearing about employee relations, budgets, the principle of supply and demand, employee counseling and communication, crisis management, and consumer relations. Responsibility and accountability were two concepts that my father drummed into my head. I remember one day wanting to call in sick to work; I was sixteen and had a part-time job in a bakery. I really wasn't ill and just wanted the night off. My father sat me down and gave me my first official lesson in employee commitment and employer dilemma. Needless to say I went to work and never quite have forgotten that valuable lesson. Business conversations were openly shared in our house, and when my brother and I became old enough our opinions were, and continued to be, welcomed regarding business matters.

A second in-house role model was my mother; she always helped my father with various aspects of clerical upkeep of the business. Her opinions were always solicited when it came to new ideas or problem-solving sessions. Here I saw true partnership in action. She was a source of support for my father. It was through my mother that I learned that a woman could be an asset to a business and that she could grasp what seemed to be complicated matters, and make a real contribution in a man's world.

So, through my parental role modeling, I received my first lessons in entrepreneurial activities and partnership interaction.

Other circumstances that may be considered contributory were that both my grandfathers came to this country in the last century and owned and operated their own businesses; one was an ice-and-coal wholesaler and the other was a barber who owned the neighborhood shop. Lastly, out of ten uncles, six of them also owned their own businesses.

Role Models: Nursing

The next group of role models that I consider important were the nurses who influenced my decision to become a nurse and my education to prepare for this role. My next-door neighbor was the first nurse I ever really knew. She was just a few years older than I was and always seemed to enjoy her work. It was at her suggestion that I considered applying to nursing school, after completion of junior college. I remember Diane stressing to me that the profession of nursing offered many opportunities for movement within its framework. Not totally convinced that nursing was for me, I got a job as an emergency room clerk at a local hospital. There I was exposed to an entire group of nurses working as a team, enjoying their work and each other. I very much liked interacting with them and soon became frustrated with my clerk job because I wanted to do more for the patients. So, in September of 1971, I entered nursing school.

Nursing school was a positive experience for me. My instructors were helpful, warm, and caring people. The director of the program was a dynamic individual. She was responsible for designing and implementing the program at the college the year before I came. She was the kind of person who had tremendous energy and was involved in many projects, yet always had time to sit and chat. While I was in school, she received the governor's appointment to chair the Board of Registered Nurses. Although she was not in business, she was an excellent role model and represented someone who had a successful career in a nontraditional nursing situation. I always found her to be stimulating and intriguing.

In my junior year as a nursing student, I was offered an opportunity to participate as a student instructor for the fundamental nursing class. This gave me the opportunity to work with women I had admired and proved to be a fruitful time for me. It was at this point that I decided that I wanted to go on to graduate school in nursing so that I could someday teach.

As I grew in my ability as a nurse, I changed. Change, though scary, has always presented a challenge for me. After almost three years of staff nursing, I began to search for more in my profession. Torn between feelings of disillusionment with nursing and a remembered desire to go to graduate school, I opted to do the most obvious thing and put off any decision for a while. Instead, I took a job as a head nurse in an outpatient gynecologic oncology clinic. There I met my very first mentor in nursing.

The dictionary defines *mentor* as a wise and faithful counselor.

My first mentor in nursing was a nursing administrator I met while in orientation for my new job. She too was in orientation and we immediately formed an alliance. She was to be my boss for the next three years. She was a strong woman with a solid commitment to nursing. She relied on me to run my clinic the best way I knew how and was there whenever I needed her. She taught me things about administration and helped me learn. She helped me to apply theory to practical nursing administration situations and gave me my first lesson in nursing politics, which proved to be a valuable asset to my career.

Risk Taking

The Chinese symbol for risk is a combination of the symbols for danger and opportunity (Winston 1979). I truly view risk as an opportunity. I have always seen myself, and have always been seen by others, as a risk taker. As early in my life as I can remember, I would run the risk of punishment or reprimand to accomplish a deliciously tempting venture I truly believed I was right in embarking on. My parents have told me stories, which I vaguely remember, about a child who just went ahead and did what she pleased; a child with a mind of her own. So, I must believe that risk-taking behavior has been with me for quite some time.

In *Skills for Success,* by Adele Scheele, a skill called *risk-linking* is discussed. Risk-linking is the ability to take a leap into the unknown and accept the consequences. It is an exploration of new experiences with which we may not feel comfortable or secure, a search for a concrete opportunity, a new direction, most noticeably practiced when there is a need for change (Scheele 1979).

Early in my career as a nurse, I began risk-linking—my job as teaching assistant, my move from staff nurse to head nurse, and a move from head nurse to supervisor. When I accepted these jobs, I was unsure of my abilities to accomplish them. I was always willing to try, succeed or fail; I didn't want to pass up an opportunity. It was through these positive experiences that I gained confidence and the ability to face new and exciting challenges. I began to develop a pattern of successful risk-linking in my profession.

The creation and the development of the business, HCFI, was just down the road a short way. Looking back, the risk was not really in the creation but in the implementation. Risk in the business is ongoing. Each time we pick up a new project or potential client, a risk exists.

Risks we continue to face result in advantages or disadvantages. Which they are considered to be is really up to the individual. I see our business risks falling into four categories: (1) financial, or the loss of our original investment; (2) failure of the business or the loss of our time and our energy; (3) role-confusion and resultant stress; and (4) success.

Role-confusion exists as we cross another transitional bridge in the vast profession of nursing. It is often stressful to function as a service-based nurse while performing duties required of us by traditional nursing jobs, then having to adjust our minds to the alternative roles of nurse-businessperson in attempting to present ourselves as competent peers in the world of entrepreneurship.

I believe that any risk presented is clearly an advantage. Succeed or fail—the experience is in the doing.

Feelings of Independence and Control

These two feelings are closely related. Once feelings of independence emerge, there's no putting them down (Winston 1979). To me, independence and control mean freedom, and freedom translates into increased ability to create.

In traditional hospital nursing, creativity can sometimes be stifled. Feelings of frustration can decrease one's energy level; the more energy spent dealing with politics and bureaucratic problems, the less energy there is to create. Creativity can be the best friend to change. More and more, hospital nursing services would certainly benefit from a little creative change.

Our health consultation business has been the creative force that has sparked enthusiasm in many of our peers who have chosen to work with us on projects. That in itself is a motivational factor for my partners and myself.

We had in mind, when developing this business, the creation of a vehicle that nurses could work through to exercise their talents as health consultants, health educators, and creative problem-solvers. We also wanted to give them full range of creative expression. Most have enjoyed their relationship with us and continue to be available for us. When they come to us disillusioned and frustrated about their careers, and leave feeling happy and optimistic about a creative future in nursing, we feel confident that our idea is working. We hope that our enterprise prospers so that we may continue to provide a vehicle for creative expression for nurses.

Resources

Everybody needs resources to succeed. Without them, a project such as the development of a business may never occur. In explaining resources, it is important to recognize that we, ourselves, were, and are, our own primary resources. We were eager and enthusiastic, and we wanted our ideas to work. We wanted to succeed. Take the diversity of our personalities and our backgrounds and add our educational expertise and our joint learning experiences, and our first-line resources come to life. By combining our own special needs, we formed the foundation upon which the business is built.

Other resources include time and commitment, without which we would have nothing. If we were serious about this business, and we were, then we had to realistically assess the amount of time each of us could willingly devote to it. We have all had to make changes in our schedules to accommodate this project in our busy lives. One thing that has been extremely helpful is that we periodically sit down and each reassess our commitment to HCFI. It is helpful to know that someone else is feeling tired, stressed, and pressured for time but is willing to continue to support a commitment.

Of course, our next most important resource was money. We were fortunate in that we had done some work and had been paid prior to our filing the incorporation papers. Therefore, the business itself actually paid for that costly situation. We each were willing to make an initial investment to cover the cost of office supplies and stationery. We also each put $25.00 a month in an office maintenance fund to cover postage, typing, and telephone expenses. We have all had to keep full- or part-time jobs so that we may support ourselves and the business upkeep.

The last resources are ones we could have never done without— our friends and relatives who believed in us and supported us from the beginning. They are truly assets to HCFI. First, there are our colleagues who are willing to work with us as independent consultants. Next, there are those outside the field of health care whose consultation assists us in the areas where our knowledge is lacking such as public relations, marketing and advertising, legal counsel, and business counsel.

Feelings of Displacement

We all became increasingly frustrated in our traditional nursing jobs, and we sought to make some changes. In looking around at what the job market and profession had to offer, we grew even more discouraged. We realized that we ourselves would have to create the next exciting and challenging experience in nursing. We were searching for greater professional and personal fulfillment. Through our combined experiences, we saw many incongruities in the health care system and felt the need to get involved. We believed that we had something to offer and that we could help change the system and make it better. We believed that only through private enterprise could we exercise future vision and possibly create workable solutions. Although we were not economically motivated, financial factors were involved. Perhaps our greatest quest in this project was to make a professional statement.

The Development of a Business: An Assessment

Late in 1978, a few friends and I talked about my idea of establishing some sort of a nursing business. Perhaps one of the most important things to look at when searching for just the right partner or partners in a business such as ours is similar philosophy. The first person I encountered in my search for comrades was Sal Esparza, a friend for many years from the old days of the Student Nurses Association. We had kept in touch since nursing school and when I approached him about the idea, his face lit up like a Christmas tree. We spent some time talking and found that our thoughts on the matter were very similar. Feeling that perhaps we might need more support in the way of a third partner, we looked for someone with a similar philosophy and found Deborah Bolton, another old friend, with whom I had worked at UCLA about two years earlier. By mid-1979, we had made the decision to put something together but we didn't know where to begin.

I was in my fourth quarter of graduate school and was taking a class called Generic Consultation. One section of the class was set aside for learning the process involved in system assessment. This section presented an excellent opportunity to learn how an outside consultant assesses an established system for problem-solving or program planning. Part of the final exam for the class was the presentation of an assessment of a working system, complete with diagram. We were to identify the system strengths and weaknesses and to make some viable suggestions about correcting the weaknesses. In the other part of the class, we learned about negotiation, contract setting, consultation scheduling, and the art of becoming a good consultant. This class was one of the most interesting and stimulating experiences of my graduate education; it was also quite useful. The system that I had originally chosen to assess had decided at the last minute to cancel. I was left in a bind, and usually when that happens the only thing left to do is to exercise resourcefulness. It was at that time that I decided to go ahead and take our ideas about health consultation and create a system.

My two partners agreed and we began to work on what seemed to be a good idea. As my preliminary research, I collected some articles that related to independent nursing practices and/or businesses. To my surprise, there had been several articles written outlining the conceptualization process, development, problem-area identification, and evaluation of a business. Other articles covered legal issues, and others discussed organizational issues and services offered. After a careful review of the articles, I met with my cohorts and in one evening we briefly sketched out a framework, philosophies, objectives, and formats for processes of interactions for what we then called Quality Health Care Consultants and what is today known as Health Communicators Foundation, Inc. We also discussed administrative strategies, organizational structure, types of client services, and functional components of the business.

Next, I took all the information and processed it, drew my diagram, and wrote up my system assessment. It was a great experience! I had full range of creativity with no limits placed on me. When the day came to present it in class, I thought to myself, "How crazy is this idea?" With a slight bit of reservation, I gave my presentation. After I was done, to my delight, they loved it. Once again, my risk-taking behavior paid off. Our ideas were supported and reinforced by our peers. My partners were excited when I told them the news. We were happy and proud of what we had created and grew strong in our commitment to take what was on paper and make it come to life.

From May to August, we met weekly to begin formalizing our plans. We fantasized and did a lot of regular old brainstorming. We consulted with our friend Janet, a nurse who owned her own registry, and taught some classes for her. I began doing some consultation with the film industry from referrals, and we even were asked to meet a group from the Rand Corporation and Northrop University. Quite a feather in our caps!

Starting small is perhaps the best advice I can give to any budding entrepreneurs. We were babes in the woods and seemed at times to get ourselves in way over our heads. Our enthusiasm and belief in both ourselves and our ideas made it possible for us to get in the door, but the ability to follow through was a problem in situations presenting a large amount of work or a lot of research. Not that it couldn't be done, but time is always an important factor to consider.

We each did some small jobs within the areas of our own clinical expertise and we continued to pursue our educational objectives and our career plans. One of the best assets that a partnership can create is that the work can be shared and each person can have the ability to continue to pursue objectives in education or career. We knew it would be a long time before the business could ever support all three of us with salaries comparable to what we might make in our chosen roles within traditional nursing. Both Debbie and I are cancer nurse specialists, having received our graduate education at UCLA, and Sal is a cardiovascular nurse specialist. Aside from our areas of clinical expertise, we present a rather varied selection of functional ability. Both Sal and I had had experience in administration and we have all prepared and lectured extensively. Presently, Sal is a nurse recruiter and Terry a nurse researcher, adding additional talents to our group. I recently enjoyed a year or so as a clinical nurse specialist; however, both Debbie and I are presently working solely through HCFI.

In early 1980, Debbie asked me to attend a showing of a new three-dimensional microscope with her. A friend of ours had suggested that the owners of the company might want to discuss some type of business interaction. We went as representatives of the business to see if there was anything that we could offer in the way of consultation. Of course, we had a few ideas that we only partially revealed; they liked our thoughts and asked for a second meeting. However, something seemed strange and I found myself feeling uncomfortable with some of the glances and comments that were being made by the company's representatives, who were men. When I looked at Debbie, I could tell that she felt the same. After this meeting, we decided to return the next day with what I like to call our secret weapon: our male partner. We did return, and the atmosphere certainly changed; they communicated on a much more professional level and Debbie and I felt more at ease.

That situation has not occurred very frequently, but when it does, we know exactly what to do. I think perhaps the reason it doesn't occur that frequently is because after almost one and a half years, Debbie and I are both more sure of ourselves and our presentation reflects that. There are still a few male chauvinists around, and when they show their true colors, it's time once again for that secret weapon.

Incorporation: Let's Make It Official

It was after that experience that the three of us made the decision to incorporate. We were going to go ahead and do some health marketing research for that company, and we thought it was time to take the final risk.

One day while visiting with a psychologist friend of ours, we started talking about projects that we might do together. He liked the idea of the business and thought that he could be an asset to us. After serious deliberation between Debbie, Sal, and myself we went ahead and looked into a legal arrangement including our psychologist friend.

We consulted our lawyer and asked if he would investigate various corporation laws and partnership agreements, although we had our minds set on incorporation. The day came for Glenn to present what his investigation had revealed.

We were told that in the state of California, nurses were not recognized as professionals; therefore, it was not possible for us to own equal shares of a professional corporation with someone who was considered a professional. If we did incorporate with the psychologist, he must own 51% of the corporation and we must split 49%, meaning that each of us would only own 16.5% of the company. We were not about to give up equal ownership of something we created, began to develop, and worked so long and hard for. The reason this law existed was then explained to us by our friend. The nonprofessional nurse should not have any evaluative mechanism over the practice of the professional, and if the nurse owned more of a percentage of the corporation than the psychologist, legally s/he would. Conversely, the professional, in this case the psychologist, would and should by law have an evaluative mechanism over the nurse. A mutual decision was reached and we excluded the psychologist from our project.

The Process

We next received information from our current attorney regarding the pros and cons of partnership versus incorporation. A for-profit corporation provides a systematic method for collecting the capital needed to open the business by allowing interested persons to purchase the stock and share in the profits. Since the corporation is considered a legal entity, individual stockholder's personal financial liability is limited to the amount of their investment. However, in most partnerships, each partner is personally liable to the extent of his net worth. The traditional corporate structure also provides a basic model for management (Zahourek 1979).

On March 26, 1980, we were recognized as a closed business corporation by the state of California. I wish I had logged the number of hours that led to that event. After three years of spent time and tremendous energy, our efforts came to fruition. We happily toasted the signing of the papers, not suspecting the amount of work that was ahead. This was truly the beginning.

Our rationale for choosing a name that did not include the word *nurse* proved to be sound. We had felt from the start that our services would and could transcend the scope of traditional nursing activities. We are not an employment registry nor a private nursing practice. Leaving the word *nurse* out of our name has not locked us into any public misconception of who or what we are or do. Our present name is well suited for what we do and we are happy with the decision.

Who Are We and What Do We Do?
Exactly what do we do and for whom do we do it? These are questions I am sure you are asking by this time. We see ourselves as consultants, providing education, counseling, and problem-solving services in the area of health. Our client services are divided into three groups and are based on the framework presented by Archer and Fleshman (1978). The areas are as follows: direct services to individual clients or groups of clients; semidirect services to health agencies, private industry, or community groups, in which we help them deliver better quality care to their clients; indirect services to those organizations who focus on the systems involved with provision of health awareness, such as private agencies, industry, and the community at large. Our fees are based on an individual project basis. Fee schedules were difficult at first. Nurses have always undervalued their services; as a result, the public rates the value of nursing in accordance (Rafferty and Carner 1973). We are beginning to feel much more comfortable about asking for fees that seem reasonable for the amount of time and energy that goes into our projects.

Initially, the board of directors of HCFI consisted of only three officers, but we recently voted to take on another member, who was brought into the company as an equal partner. Our board consists of a president (myself) and three vice-presidents. The board is responsible for all aspects of business management. Sal is the vice-president in charge of finance and he keeps the financial records, pays the bills, and confers with our accountant on fiscal matters. Debbie is the vice-president in charge of correspondence, she keeps the minutes of the meetings, a state requirement, and takes care of other general correspondence. Terry Chamarro, our third and newest member, is still getting used to the business itself and we have not clearly decided on her specific functions. As president, I am responsible for quality assurance of projects, programs, and individual consultants; however, a high degree of individual accountability is stressed as we seek help from one another and outside consultants on our projects.

Each officer is also responsible for finding his or her own projects either through referral or solicitation. That person then becomes the project coordinator responsible for direct negotiation and communication with the contracting agent or agency. The coordinator is responsible for all project budget proposals and financial arrangements; each project has a zero-based budget. The project coordinator must bring all matters to the board for a three-fourths vote to pass any decision.

The board of directors meets bimonthly. Because of our busy schedules, we found it necessary to block off meeting times six months in advance and commit ourselves to being there. After general business is discussed, each individual project coordinator gives an update on the project's progress and may also bring any problems or concerns to the board's attention for a vote or for consultation. The project coordinator may choose to use a fellow board member as a coordinator or may choose an outside consultant, based on specialty need. That coordinator is contracted to HCFI and negotiates a fee with us. We then will contract with the agent or agency we are providing the service for. Contracts have become a very important part of our business transactions because we have at times used three- and four-party transactions. Responsibility for public relations, marketing, and advertising also rests with the project coordinator.

The Human Side of Partnership

As you can see, we use the group process in all our business interactins, especially when decision making is called for. In the beginning, partnership meant support and it still does. It was scary being a nurse interested in pursuing a business. Safety and support came when I found others around me who thought and felt the same and wanted to share in this risky endeavor. Being in a business partnership is something like being in a marriage. It is also like being a small family unit. In looking at the theory of family homeostasis, we have gotten a better understanding of how we function and support one another. When we are all in town and everyone is functioning at their normal levels of activity, all is well and we are in a balanced homeostatic condition. If one person, who may be a project coordinator or in the midst of a negotiation, goes out of town or is under a tremendous amount of stress, then any of the others take over so that the homeostatic balance will not be threatened.

Through our interactions we have learned to trust one another. We have learned one another's strengths and weaknesses. We have seen each other angry and upset and we have seen each other fail and succeed. We have helped each other many times by listening and by sharing our feelings.

One of the first experiences of our partnership came prior to our first business meeting with the Rand Corporation. A few days before the meeting, we sat down to discuss how we might interact at that meeting. First we took a look at what our best and most natural skills were, then we focused on how these worked together to our advantage. For example, we were each given a role to perform then and during our business meeting with Rand. Debbie was the initiator, Sal the observer, and I the interpreter. In a sense, we were smart to bring our best talents to awareness so each of us knew what the other was doing. Not having ever interacted together in a group with others, we actually were rehearsing.

Recently, at a business meeting we had, I sat back and watched the interaction of the three of us. Again, I saw those same three roles being played. This time, however, there was no prior discussion or rehearsal—we were just doing what came naturally.

Partnership can be a rewarding experience. It does require a great deal of work. The secret to a successful partnership is threefold: Trust, open communication, and a genuine interest in each other—truly a human experience.

The Future

It is very hard to tell at this point just where Health Communicators is going. I do know that we have an incredible amount of potential, and with our continued commitment and hard work, the sky is the limit. My partners share these feelings with me and display equal amounts of enthusiasm. The support that we have built around us also fortifies us and keeps us optimistic that HCFI may be around for a long time.

I truly feel that the essence of success in any type of business is vision. Vision to see and feel what the future holds. As Toffler (1970) has shown us, change is a dynamic process that continues to occur at a dizzying pace. Change occurs to all things. The ability to move with change in a planned, systematic way requires vision. Considering the scope of future vision, we at HCFI must look at many factors—for example, the changes in governmental control of health care (as a right instead of a privilege) and the type of role the consumer may choose to take in his or her own health care (active or traditionally passive). The overall economy of the nation is also extremely important and must be considered if any business wishes to survive. Last, but most important, are the changes that continue to bombard the nursing profession. We must keep a keen eye on all these changes and try to stay a bit ahead of them in both our awareness and our planning. That is what will keep HCFI viable and challenging for its creators.

Because we have not chosen to limit our scope of services, it has been easy for us to branch out. We will continue this branching out and take advantage of any project that presents a health issue within it. We believe in ourselves and in our profession's ability to meet the challenges of the future and assist in making dynamic changes in health care today.

We are proud of what we have built, and possess a great sense of pride in our accomplishments.

References

Archer, Sarah E., and Fleshman, Ruth. "Doing Our Own Thing: Community Health Nurses in Independent Practice." *Journal of Nursing Administration,* 8(11):44-51, November 1978.

Rafferty, Rita, and Carner, Jean. "Nursing Consultants Incorporated: A Corporation." *Journal of Nursing Administration,* 21 (4):2 232-235, April 1973.

Scheele, Adele. *Skills for Success.* New York: William Morrow, 1979.

Toffler, Alvin. *Future Shock.* New York: Random House, 1970.

Winston, Sandra. *The Entrepreneurial Woman.* New York: Bantam, 1979.

Zahourek, Rothlyn. "Two Management Systems in a Nursing Private Practice Group." *Journal of Nursing Administration,* 9 (9):48-51, September 1979.

Bibliography

Agree, Betty. "Beginning an Independent Nursing Practice." *American Journal of Nursing* 74(4):636-624, April 1974.

Keller, Nancy. "The Evolution of a Successful Partnership." *Journal of Nursing Administration,* 7(8):6-9, 35, October 1977.

Kaltz, Charles J. *Private Practice in Nursing.* Germantown, Maryland: Aspen Systems Corp., 1979.

Zahourek, Rothlyn; Leone, Delores; and Long, Frank. *Creative Health Services: A Model for Group Nursing Practice.* St. Louis: Mosby, 1976.

3

Joint Practice with a Physician

Shirley St. Amand

"Persons who are growth-motivated try to increase their own potential. They view growth as fulfillment—the degree of measure of at-
taining one's desired end-success" (Spengler and Grissum 1976,
p. 268). Growth-motivated individuals are usually goal-oriented.
Growth through goal-orientation has been the major force in my
nursing career. Leaving a conventional hospital setting to establish
my own consulting business as a cardiology nurse practitioner can be
viewed as the culmination of years of planning short- and long-term
professional goals.

Two years of working in an acute care setting in Boston proved to
be a turning point in my career. Part of being a nursing professional
means being accountable, having direct influence in the decision-
making process for patient care, and having the freedom to practice
nursing. The acute care setting provided little opportunity for nursing professionalism. The everyday drudgery of task-oriented nursing,
the lack of respect from physicians, and a general feeling of powerlessness made me realize the need to plot a specific professional
course. The alternative would be a career plagued by frustration.

My reading in professional nursing journals showed me that some
nurses were doers and innovators. Their involvement seemed to be
molding the future of nursing. As one who thrived on responsibility,
autonomy, and professionalism, I began to recognize that the only

way I could become a doer and innovator would be to seek nursing independence outside the setting of a major acute care institution. I decided to leave the hospital and branch out into the community. This became my opportunity for growth and my primary long-term goal.

Before pursuing this alternative, however, I needed more formal education. Since I was a diploma graduate, this meant acquiring a bachelor of science in nursing (BSN) degree. Leaving the hospital setting to enroll at the university was a risk that demonstrated my determination to advance professionally. The university milieu rekindled my zeal for nursing and strengthened my commitment to being successful. I earned my BSN degree and immediately planned ahead.

As an undergraduate I had become acquainted with the new concept of a master's-prepared nurse practitioner. I had read enthusiastically about the successes of such forerunners of the nurse practitioner movement as Lucille Kinlein in independent practice in Virginia and Kathleen Brown in private practice with a group of physicians in Maryland. Suddenly, this new dimension in nursing seemed to be exactly what I had been searching for. Well prepared to work in an autonomous role in the community and having the power to define their practice, these master's-degree graduates represented a new era in the profession of nursing.

I now regarded my BSN degree as only an intermediate step toward my long-term goal of nursing independence. I became increasingly convinced that my nursing career would be based on the nurse practitioner model. However, obtaining a master's degree so soon after my BSN was financially infeasible. I was further demoralized by my projections of how long it would take to implement my new role. I estimated it might take five years after graduate school to begin to function autonomously, perhaps another five years to find an associateship with a physician who had similar professional goals. Nonetheless, I felt my long-term goal was worthwhile. If it seemed remote and out of focus, I would concentrate on a set of interim goals to sustain me.

In the short term how could I best prepare for eventual independent practice? First, it was clear that I had to return to school for a master's degree in order to firmly establish my academic credentials. I resolved to do this within three years. Second, during this three-year period I intended to familiarize myself with a variety of nursing roles and models in order to acquire a solid nursing foundation. This would be critical in achieving and maintaining nursing autonomy. In pursuit of this goal I became an instructor in a hospital-based nursing diploma program. This position afforded me the opportunity to study and present diverse nursing points of view in a methodical and scholarly way.

My goal of entering graduate school in a nurse practitioner program was realized on schedule. I was fortunate enough to be accepted into a highly regarded program and motivated enough to relocate from Pennsylvania to California to enroll. Once enrolled, I was not content to let the course of study supplant my personal goal-setting. I had always worked in the cardiovascular field and I wanted to concentrate my studies in cardiology. My dream was to join a cardiology private practice. When the school of nursing offered me a semester preceptorship in an emergency room, I argued that it was inconsistent with my goals. How was I to become proficient in cardiology while working in a setting with no long-term follow-up care? How many emergency cases would be cardiac related? On my own initiative I arranged for a cardiology preceptorship in a setting where I would be exposed to a range of cardiac problems. Not only did this adjustment bring me closer to my goals, it served to enhance my future marketability as a nurse practitioner.

Similarly, my personal goal-setting helped me to decide in favor of writing a thesis rather than sitting for the customary comprehensive exams. I had developed an interest in research and believed that an understanding of research methodology would be invaluable for an independent nursing practice. My thesis research project proved to be a significant educational experience made possible by proper goal-setting.

Setting Up Independent Practice

Nursing's image is frequently linked with powerlessness. Many factors contribute to this powerlessness. One factor is legislative inconsistency. In some states, nurses in hospitals are not allowed to practice nursing as defined by their state nursing practice laws because of other state regulations governing the operation of acute care settings. Another factor is the relationship between power and the generation of revenue in hospitals. Physicians generate hospital revenue, although their personal income is derived independently. Nurses, on the other hand, generate no direct hospital revenue and their wages are derived from patient room and board. As a result, hospital administrators empower physicians by becoming dependent upon them. When hospital priorities are established, nurses' needs are invariably secondary to those of physicians.

Nurses as employees are automatically cast in a subservient role. This disadvantage causes nurses as individuals to lose some of the autonomy nursing as a profession would normally maintain. I began to realize that nurses would never have the same status as physicians until they demonstrated a similar capacity to generate revenue for services rendered. Money is a powerful lever. In the case of nursing, it can lead the way to autonomy.

As I began to refine my thoughts on finding and joining a cardiology practice, this insight into the dynamics of power, money, and autonomy convinced me that I would have to be financially independent in any business arrangement. This meant being an independent consultant rather than a salaried associate. I would establish fees for service or negotiate for a percentage of the practice revenues. I would share a portion of the monthly overhead expenses to allow me legitimate access to office space, secretarial assistance, office supplies, and the answering service. This strategy would avoid the imbalance of power in an employer-employee relationship. As the physician's colleague and peer, I would have the power and independence to control my practice of nursing, provide input to the joint practice, and implement change as necessary.

Of course, this was only one side of the issue. In planning for an autonomous practice, I also had to acknowledge a concomitant responsibility. I realized that promoting such a new and unfamiliar nursing role would require me to perform at a level consistent with my demands. I was prepared to accept unconventional hours, unusual patient demands, emotional involvement, as well as office management chores, business development needs, and other burdens of the practice.

Presenting such a concept to a physician with the intent of persuading him to enter into a joint practice required that I be able to demonstrate clearly the objective benefits of having a nurse practitioner in the practice. I also wanted to be able to outline definite goals for the proposed joint practice, goals that were perhaps beyond the physician's own capability. Finally, I wanted to assure myself that I was thoroughly prepared to answer questions on the definition of nurse practitioners' roles, the acceptability of nurse practitioners in various settings, the extent of malpractice coverage of expanded nursing roles, the scope of the state's nursing practice act, and the eligibility of nurse practitioners for third-party reimbursement.

After fully rehearsing my conceptual framework, I wanted to be able to demonstrate how I could be beneficial to a particular practice. Certain situations would be more viable than others. I had to ask certain questions. Is the practice mainly office hours with little hospital involvement, or is it mainly hospital rounds with few office hours? Is it a new practice or an established practice? Where is the practice located? If it was in an affluent community with an abundance of physicians, I knew the chances of joint practice acceptability would be less than in a mixed socioeconomic community.

At this point I looked to the future. I was confident that I had taken all reasonable measures to prepare for joint practice. Within only a few months of obtaining my master's degree I was referred to a physician who had been considering bringing a nurse practitioner into his practice. He had been in successful solo practice for seven years. The practice had grown to the point where one person could not manage it comfortably. Although he was looking for an associate, he was not looking for another physician. A nurse associate would be more in keeping with his vision of providing total patient care while maintaining the practice at a constant size.

It was apparent that we were philosophically compatible. We began the long process of communicating our thoughts. We placed special emphasis on exchanging our short- and long-term personal and professional goals since they would become the basis of how we would define our practice. Both of us had similar primary goals: the need to be active in the academic community, the desire to do clinical research, and, most important, the commitment to deliver quality patient care. We also took care to explain our special needs and role expectations in order to avoid future misunderstanding.

The physician accepted my contention that only the broadest possible definition of my role would truly allow me to achieve my professional goals. I defined a role with three principal components: clinical practice, teaching, and clinical research and writing. Clinical practice would encompass seeing patients in the office, making hospital rounds, making home visits as necessary, holding individual counseling sessions, leading group educational sessions, and undertaking any other projects to improve quality care. Teaching would involve guest lecturing to university students and hospital nurses. Clinical research and writing would consist of statistically documenting our treatment programs, and publishing articles in nursing and medical journals. We both recognized that this role would require flexible hours that would have to be balanced against the daily needs of the practice.

Risk taking is inherent in developing a new role. This became evident when I pursued the point of being an independent consultant rather than a salaried employee. Devising an unconventional financial relationship would be a risk for both of us.

Receptive to new and creative ideas, the physician was open to my suggestion of payment on a contractual basis. Since we both would be involved to varying degrees in every facet of the practice, we decided it would be too complicated to determine our individual compensation based on separate fees for our combined services. We agreed that I would receive a constant percentage of the monthly office revenues from the activities in which I was specifically involved. I would receive no fee for activities such as the physician's contracted services in the hospital. We chose a percentage that represented a fair personal income based on an analysis of the office revenues of the practice. Obviously, my monthly income would vary according to the number of patients seen and the status of the accounts receivable.

This arrangement seemed workable. However, since we did not know each other's professional capabilities, I suggested that we work together for three months with the option of strengthening or dissolving the association after that time. This agreement allowed both of us the opportunity to assess our basic compatibility and our professional styles.

Implementation of the Role

My role has evolved as originally planned. I am not confined to a small segment of the practice; rather, I am totally involved in every aspect. I see patients in the office, both new consultations and follow-up patients. As individual problems arise, I arrange special counseling sessions to help meet that patient's needs. These counseling sessions involve diet, conflict in personal interrelationships, risk-factor modification, and stress management. I have started group sessions in the office to deal with patient weight reduction.

Every day I make rounds with my physician associate at the two hospitals where we provide concurrent nursing and medical input for our hospitalized patients. My nursing input is particularly important because patients continue to need care for their chronic problems after being admitted to the hospital for an acute problem. As necessary, I make home visits after discharge to assess the patient's progress. In general, my ability to detect health problems or to progress a patient more quickly than expected has saved the patient both money and further illness or injury.

I also support and contribute to the hospital nursing programs. I make nursing rounds with the nurses so that they see that I operate from a nursing framework and that I am really a nurse practitioner and not a "mini-physician." I lecture in their critical care courses and have been working closely with nursing service in setting up guidelines for nurse practitioner hospital privileges.

Strengths and Limitations of Joint Practice

Having been in practice with a physician for three years, I am now able to reflect on the strengths and limitations of this unique enterprise. I was very privileged to join a practice that had been well established for seven years. This afforded me full and equal access to an established clientele. Fortunately, if a patient objected to the team concept my associate was able to accept the loss of that business if necessary. Even office space was no problem since my associate's suite was large enough to accommodate another office.

Our initial wide-ranging discussions about goals and values have been instrumental in helping us cope with the inevitable stress and strain of a professional relationship. For example, when our patients pose questions to each of us independently to test how synchronized we are in our program of care, we take great pride in knowing that they will receive the same response from us both. Our continuing mutual respect and compatibility have allowed us to maximize our strengths and professional growth. We never feel that either of us spends too much time with outside professional activities or that either is not functioning as the other deems appropriate.

I have found it essential to continuously educate those around me about the nurse practitioner role. This holds true not only for health personnel at all levels within the hospital, but for my physician associate as well. I regularly give him journal articles on nurse practitioners and keep him abreast of developments in the nurse practitioner movement. The nursing orientation I have provided serves to assist him in defining my role to his colleagues and other medical groups.

My strong nursing background has proved to be extremely helpful. Defining my role strictly from the nursing perspective has allayed much fear and anxiety within both the medical and the nursing communities. My offering to speak on nursing philosophies and frameworks has done more for the advancement of this progressive role than the actual implementation of the role itself.

Actual implementation of the nurse practitioner role has brought many frustrations. Perhaps the greatest frustration has been the inability to obtain hospital privileges at the institutions where we make our daily rounds. Eighty percent of our practice is hospital-based. We predicated our joint practice on my having independent access to our hospitalized patients. At the time we established our joint practice, the medical bylaws of one particular institution did not allow nurses to obtain hospital privileges. Ever since I submitted my application for privileges two and a half years ago, I have worked with the joint practice committee to help establish some mechanism for processing and evaluating nurse practitioner applicants. Recently, the medical bylaws were changed to allow nurse practitioners to apply for hospital privileges. Consequently, I have temporary privileges and expect a permanent appointment as soon as the Board of Directors votes on it.

Another frustration is the lack of full acceptance of my role by my nursing colleagues in the hospital. I am not part of the institution or its politics. I wear a lab coat, not a uniform. Because of my association with a physician, nurses frequently perceive only that aspect of my role that overlaps with medicine rather than that aspect of my role that derives from nursing. In order to counter such misperceptions I have made it a point to have direct personal contact with members of the nursing staff so that I could assure them of my role as an independent nurse practitioner. I feel that with time the role will be better understood.

A similar frustration is lack of peer support. There are very few nurse practitioners in the community who have their own business in a clinical practice setting. I recognize that peer critique and collaboration are important for the long-term success of my role. In order to fill the void of peer support in the community, I am active in the Nurse Practitioner Special Interest Group of the State Nurses' Association. I also maintain a dialogue with colleagues in related professions. The principal need, however, is to continuously reevaluate the effectiveness of the role in the context of our daily practice. The day-to-day demands of the practice are so pressing that effective role implementation requires a constant reassessment of how the role can better meet the needs of the patients, the practice, and my own goals.

Lack of time has proved to be a major factor in preventing me from readily achieving my goal for writing and publishing. It has been very difficult to collect my thoughts and write after working twelve to fifteen hours a day, six or seven days a week. To generate support for this endeavor, I decided to start a small writing group composed of nurses interested in publishing. The writing group has been a good forum for exchanging information on writing techniques, writing research, and the procedure for dealing with publishers. Since founding the group I have submitted manuscripts of chapters for two new books on nursing.

A final source of frustration has been my own lack of business education and experience. Being an independent practitioner means being self-employed. Successful implementation of the nurse practitioner role as I have defined it depends on my running a successful business. As part of my initiation into the business world, I had to hire a tax consultant to help me project yearly earnings, depreciate office equipment, and identify tax-deductible expenses. I had to familiarize myself with the requirements for payment of quarterly federal and state income taxes, the state self-employment tax, city business tax, and state disability premium. I also came to realize how much extra income I needed to generate in order to compensate for the loss of standard employee benefits such as prepaid health insurance, retirement plan, sick leave, and holidays.

Running a successful business requires effective management skills and techniques. Knowing how to relate to office personnel and deal with daily office problems is invaluable. In order to maximize the effectiveness of the office and help ensure open communication among the office personnel, we have instituted a monthly business meeting away from the office. These meetings allow for individual input regarding office problems and policies in a relaxed and detached environment.

My involvement in the management of the practice has given me a special opportunity to witness the installation of a computer data processing system that helps us with our billing, record keeping, and other office tasks. I am eager to become knowledgeable about a system that will revolutionize the future of the health care industry.

Another new learning experience has been investigating different aspects of relocating our office to another part of the city. Planning such a move has forced me to deal with factors that the mainstream of nursing never considers. My evaluations of possible locations, the cost of renting versus buying, renovation costs, new equipment purchases, and projections of office growth served to remind me how important planning is to a practice.

My perception of the strengths and limitations of joint practice is interwoven with my personal philosophy of growth-orientation and goal-setting. The limitations tend to be conditions or events that thwart growth and achievement of goals. The strengths tend to be conditions or events that facilitate growth and achievement of goals. My primary goal has always been professionalism and autonomy in my nursing career. At this point in time, I am close to achieving that goal. I have my own business. I practice autonomously. I define the role to suit my needs, personality, and future goals. I can initiate new projects and programs. I can effect change. Most of all, I am free to grow with the practice and the profession.

Future Possibilities

Three years has been a relatively short period of time for full implementation of this role in the community. I look forward to developing even more of an independent role as a cardiovascular nurse practitioner with direct referrals from the community. I and other nurses continue to have difficulty obtaining third-party reimbursement. I anticipate increasingly successful lobbying efforts in this matter. As of January 1980, California state law allows nonmedical personnel to incorporate with a physician. I now have the option of incorporating with my physician associate or self-incorporating. Public recognition of the independent nurse practitioner role is growing. I have received a young business leader award from the Los Angeles Junior Chamber of Commerce.

Three years in joint practice has shown that this type of professional arrangement is feasible and worth pursuing. I am enthusiastic about the seemingly limitless possibilities of my role within the practice. Despite many obstacles, I am confident that with proper growth-motivation and goal-orientation, nurse practitioners will advance to the forefront of health care delivery in the near future.

Reference

Spengler, C., and Grissum, M. *Womanpower and Health Care.* Boston: Little, Brown, 1976.

Bibliography

Brown, Kathleen. "The Nurse Practitioner in a Private Group Practice." *Nursing Outlook,* February 1974.

Jacox, Ada, and Norris, Catherine. *Organizing for Independent Nursing Practice.* New York: Appleton-Century-Crofts, 1977.

Kinlein, Lucille. *Independent Nursing Practice with Clients.* Philadelphia: Lippincott, 1977.

Koltz, Charles, Jr. *Private Practice in Nursing.* Rockville, Maryland: Aspen Systems Corporation, 1979.

Mundinger, M. *Autonomy in Nursing.* Rockville, Maryland: Aspen Systems Corporation, 1980.

4

Publishing:
The National Nursing Review

Christopher M. Smith
Sandra F. Smith

Question: Tell me about the National Nursing Review.
Sandra: We are in the business of nursing education. Specifically, we publish and market review textbooks for nursing students who are preparing for the RN or PN licensure examinations, and we conduct five-day review courses for candidates for the RN state board examinations.
Chris: Our horizons have widened lately. To our core activities we have added a series of stress management audio cassettes and a continuing education seminar. Our first book for professional nurses is under way.

Question: What led up to forming your own business and why did you take this formidable step?
Chris: Every new business has its own set of special circumstances and certainly ours was no exception. As I recall, the determining factors in our case were opportunity, necessity, and determination.
Sandra: In 1973, a teaching colleague and I conducted a psychiatric nursing review for foreign students who had great difficulty passing this part of the state board examinations. One day we asked

ourselves, "If this works for foreign nurses, why not for US graduates?" The answer to this question launched our new business and we began with one review course in northern California. We were pleased and rather amazed at the response. The next year we expanded to conducting four reviews in four different parts of the country.

Question: Were you and your partner in this business alone or were others involved as well?
Sandra: My partner and I were supported both in attitude and work by our respective husbands. My partner's husband was an attorney and Chris was a self-employed management consultant. It's important to note that all four of us had our own jobs and careers; perhaps even more crucial, we had four incomes. We all believed that there was an excellent opportunity to expand upon the original concept by adding more review sites and by producing a better nursing review book than was currently available.
Chris: We all agreed on the overall opportunity, but there arose many disagreements among us concerning just how we would develop, expand, organize, and distribute responsibilities and accountabilities. The differences over how to publish a review book—self-publishing versus contracting with an established textbook publisher—became so great that there appeared to be neither the means nor the mechanics to continue developing the business within the existing partnership relationship.

Question: You had reached your first serious crisis. How did you proceed to resolve it?
Sandra: Early in 1976, Chris and I made three very big decisions: (1) to dissolve the faltering partnership, (2) to incorporate our own business venture, and (3) to publish our own review book. My part-time teaching position at San Jose State University allowed me to devote a substantial portion of my time to organizing a team of contributing authors and to editing and formatting their material.
Chris: My schedule of consulting projects was reasonably flexible, so I had a great deal of control over my time, too. My involvement with several publishing companies and with my own independent projects provided us with contacts for such work as typesetting, paste-up, and graphic design.

Question: You've described opportunity and necessity. Now what did you mean by determination?

Sandra: Determination has been a strong factor from the beginning. We've been very motivated to make our business a success, to perform well in a competitive environment, and to provide high-quality products and services to our clientele. After all, we are in the business of helping people achieve a goal that is essential for their professional career and important from a personal standpoint.

Chris: To summarize, Sandra and I did not plan to start a business together. We each had our own independent careers, which merged because of opportunity and necessity. Once we cut loose from shore and began to row into the main current, we were very determined to "keep the ship afloat" and to develop a profitable and rewarding business.

Question: What has happened to your business, and how do these results compare to your expectations?

Sandra: The business has been far more successful than we originally envisioned. Of course, we had no experience or history on which to base a comparison. We really did not know what to expect.

Chris: The business grew rapidly because our first review book gained a significant share of the market and our review courses received an enthusiastic response. We had not drawn up a specific set of goals and schedules but we had an overall direction—growth—and a primary focus—review books and courses for RN state boards. We kept our focus on our specialty and moved as rapidly as we could to develop a solid base that would allow us to grow in the future.

Sandra: The result of the original partnership fiasco was intense competition in the existing review cities where both companies (my former partner had formed her own review company) felt they had a stake in a good market. In June 1976, we conducted reviews in San Francisco, Worcester, Mass., Los Angeles, and New York City. Within four years we had expanded to twenty-one sites in thirteen states. Over 10,000 students have attended the National Nursing Review's courses. One element in any new business that marks its success is the ability to take risks. Rather than consolidating and increasing our review locations very gradually and safely, we elected to branch out and expand as fast as possible and let the mechanisms to support this expansion catch up. In the beginning we did much of the work ourselves with part-time employees, limited office space, and limited resources, rather than making a big investment in personnel and equipment. This strategy proved to be successful, for we have recently installed a small computer.

Chris: We are now operating in a very competitive environment. Several organizations, including the parent firm of a major nursing magazine, conduct courses on a national basis. Many, many schools offer state board reviews for their own students and often for students from nearby schools. The school-sponsored sessions are usually considerably cheaper than ours and therefore tend to attract students with limited financial resources. In addition, individual nursing instructors or small groups offer courses on a local basis. We believe that the reason we keep attracting students with all of today's competition is that our reputation for quality, consistency, and an effective review has been passed along by course attendees. We carefully select our lecturers and we try to integrate only one or two new ones each year as they are needed for our expansion.

Question: You've described your review courses. What about your books?

Sandra: When people involved in book publishing ask me, "How long did it take you to put your first book together?" they are absolutely floored when I tell them that it took four and a half months. From New Year's Day, when I started telephoning prospective contributing authors, to the day we sent the manuscript to the book manufacturer (income tax day—April 15), only fourteen weeks elapsed. It took four weeks for production and by May 15 we were shipping the first copies of the 430-page first edition of *Review of Nursing for State Board Examinations.* The incredibly short production time for this book is another indication of goal accomplishment when the people involved are highly motivated and very determined to make it work. We knew that if this book was not in the bookstores by May we would miss almost an entire year of potential sales. And other publishers would have more time to publish competing books. The incentive to produce was obvious.

Question: What made you certain that you could break into the book publishing business and actually succeed.

Sandra: In making our decision to publish our own review text we thoroughly examined the factors necessary to compete in the business of publishing. The primary impetus to initiate a self-publishing business rather than go the more traditional route of big-business publishing was a sense of confidence in the book we wanted to publish and the desire to have complete control over its content, timing, production, and manufacturing. It was obvious that we would have to surrender much of this control to a publisher. This element—the strong desire to take control of one's own life—became paramount in making the decision to go ahead on our own. The second factor that influenced our decision was confidence that we had the credibility to complete the project. It is essential when one is forging ahead in an independent project to believe in the feasibility of the business. Our two career patterns and special skills needed for the business interfaced perfectly. All that remained were the resources to begin. These resources were garnered from a variety of sources including a loan from parents.

Question: How did you accomplish the feat of such a short publishing cycle?

Chris: We had twelve contributing authors sending material to us, some typed but much of it in handwritten form. With the help of a free-lance editor/proofreader, Sandra formatted, edited, and proofed the entire manuscript. We had two typesetters, a graphic designer and, at one time, three paste-up people working on the project. The excellent job of all the free-lance personnel plus the manufacturing capabilities of Kingsport Press (a former employer of mine) made it possible for us to get our own review book on the market for the June 1976 review season.

Sandra: Thus, we come to still another factor in achieving a successful outcome—planning and securing the necessary support services to assist you with your project. Our new endeavor, like most new projects, did not give us the time to develop in-house support people or services. Knowing what you need and spending adequate time to seek out these resources pays off. When it became time to use free-lance people, we made sure they were available, dependable, and predictable.

Question: What about competition in the book publishing area?

Chris: Between mid-1976 and 1980, new nursing review books (or new editions of existing ones) were published by Addison-Wesley; Arco; Lippincott; Little, Brown; Mosby; Prentice-Hall; and Pre-Test. In 1979, we expanded *Review of Nursing* to 525 pages. Our research indicates that our book was the best-selling nursing review test in the United States during the 1979-1980 academic year.

Question: What other books have you published?

Sandra: Practice Tests for State Board Examinations, published in 1978, was the result of feedback from students attending our reviews who said that they'd completed all the questions in *Review of Nursing,* and asked if we couldn't supply more. In late 1979, to make sure that we didn't let too much grass grow under our feet, we put together a team of LVN/PN teachers who submitted manuscript copy, which we published as *Review of Practical Nursing for State Board Examinations.* This book turned out to be 425 pages. Soon after this we doubled the size of *Practice Tests* and, with contributions from twenty authors, published the 430-page second edition in the fall of 1980. The business has developed far greater than our expectations, at least in this relatively short time. From a very difficult start in early 1976 to now, we have published nearly 2000 pages of manuscript material, sold over 125,000 books, and given our review courses to over 12,000 students. Our annual revenues exceed $500,000. After paying our book manufacturing costs, review expenses, and office overhead, we have had enough funds remaining to pay ourselves reasonable salaries. Also, we now have a company pension/profit-sharing plan in which all employees participate.

Question: How did you get a new business operating and still have time to arrange for such extras as fringe benefit programs?
Sandra: This brings up another important point for those starting their own businesses. When a new business is just getting off the ground there is no time to think ahead to pension-profit plans, retirement programs, or insurance and medical reimbursement plans. As soon as the day-to-day running is under control, it is important to investigate and formulate plans for integrating these aspects into the business. A common difficulty that most new businesses face is that the owners spend all their time starting new projects and trying to generate enough cash flow. They pay little or no attention to financial planning or taxes.
Chris: Two very necessary elements of any business are financial accounting and financial protection. The first, accounting, is mandatory for tax reporting, regardless of whether you operate as a partnership or a corporation. The second element, financial protection, relates to various insurance policies you need to protect yourself in the event of accident or illness. As an employee of a university, hospital, or other organization, you have various protection devices provided for you. As owner of your own business you have to protect yourself, your family, and your employees in the same manner.

Find a good accountant and a good insurance broker or agent. Ones who specialize in serving small businesses are recommended. Personal friends generally are not.

Question: What experience did you gain in your career that helped you in getting your new business launched successfully?
Sandra: My academic experience was nearly ideal to prepare me for my roles as book editor and review course coordinator. With my basic BS from Skidmore College, and master's degrees in psychiatric nursing and public health from the University of California, San Francisco, I had a reasonably broad exposure to nursing education. As a faculty member at UCSF, a consultant for California State Hospitals and New York Cornell Medical Center, and then teacher at San Jose State, I gained valuable experience in dealing with students and their needs as well as preparing and presenting curriculum content. When lecturing at state board reviews, I had many students ask me about review books. I assessed the books presently available, decided what the "ideal" book should contain, and how this material could be presented in an efficient manner. This became the formula we followed. Student response to the books has validated these theories. When you start your own business, you certainly receive much experience in a short time. I think that it is important to reflect on this experience and to be open to learning from it. A very emotional or personal approach to one's own business can narrow your focus and cause you to become inflexible. Another important aspect of having your own business is to consider options. When one approach doesn't work, try another and always keep your options open and viable.
Chris: Experience and timing are two really essential factors to consider when starting your own business. I had two years of business school at Stanford University, nine years of corporate experience, and two years of independent work. My corporate assignments in sales, marketing, planning, and public relations were invaluable, as was the more formal training at business school in accounting, finance, economics, computer sciences, and other areas. All my business experience has related to the graphic arts industry: publishing, printing, paper, graphic design, and so forth. My two years at Kingsport Press resulted in my learning quite a lot about book manufacturing and I also gained a good exposure to textbook publishing. Timing was important in my case because, as an independent consultant, I was able to allocate time and effort as needed to

work with Sandra. When our business began to grow, I cut down on my consulting work to meet the new demands of National Nursing Review. Market timing is very important also. The market was ready for a new review book. Student feedback from our early reviews indicated that graduating students would continue to respond to our course concepts as well. In summary, it is very important that your availability and the market need occur at the same time.

Question: What about a spouse as a business partner?
Sandra: In our case, our career and business experiences are very complementary, whereas our temperaments and personality traits tend to be opposites. This is a good combination because we tend to want to specialize in different aspects of the business and we do not run into many conflicts. For example, I handle the selection and management of the review lecturers and book authors. I am responsible for the contents of the books, whereas Chris is responsible for managing the production and marketing of the final product.
Chris: Many people tell us that they absolutely could not be in business with their spouses. If opportunity, necessity, and determination arrived on their doorstep, then perhaps their assessment would change. At any rate, relatively few businesses outside retail stores, restaurants, and motels are managed by husband-wife teams.
Sandra: An absolutely necessary ingredient in our success formula is a mutual respect between partners for each other's areas of responsibility while maintaining an ability to exchange constructive criticism of each other. It is difficult *always* to keep one's perspective focused on the business when strong personalities are involved, but you have to keep trying.

Question: What's the outlook for National Nursing Review?
Chris: It is clear that state board nursing review courses are accepted by the student nurses. Despite continued opposition on the part of many nursing educators (faculty, department heads, etc.), students will attend those reviews that have the reputation for providing a valuable and effective service. The competition in the review field will continue to be very strong: probably it will intensify. In July 1982 the new format for state boards will be introduced. Our review books, as well as our review courses, will be updated to conform to the new boards.
Sandra: We are not limited to state boards, however. We have expertise in gathering and presenting information for the nursing profes-

sion. To balance our present business we are exploring other ventures such as continuing education courses and books for professional nurses. Our initial CE event was a one-day seminar in San Francisco entitled "Managing Stress in the 80s." We expect to publish our first professional book within several months. Our stress management audio tapes are on the market now. So, as you can see, we are under way and moving into some closely related businesses by applying a major resource—our contributing-author/review-lecturer team—to new projects in the new markets.

Question: What advice do you have for someone who wants to publish her own book?

Sandra: Publishing a book is a more complicated project than most people realize. There are many, many steps and each must be accomplished in the proper sequence. The first step is to be clear about your objectives. What is the purpose of your proposed book? You should consider writing a prospectus just as if you were submitting the project to a major publisher. Once you have clarified your thinking and planned the entire book, write a few sample chapters. Then find a professional book editor who will act as a consultant and who will assist you in developing your manuscript. Editors perform an essential function in the publishing cycle. We would never publish material without having this outside perspective and technical advice. The more extensive editing jobs will require a development editor, while the less extensive jobs will need a copy editor.

Chris: The publishing process does not stop with the editorial steps. The two additional phases are production and marketing. Production includes design, page layout, typesetting and proofing, paste-up, and then printing and binding. There are many decisions to be made at each of these steps. Marketing the books is very important because books really do not sell themselves. You may sell a few copies to professional associates or, if you are teaching, to your students. However, achieving national distribution is entirely different. Your main avenues are (1) selling directly to the end user via direct mail, (2) selling to retail outlets, or (3) utilizing the services of a book wholesaler. National Nursing Review uses all three methods and each has its merits and problems. A fundamental problem for book publishers is the necessity of actually producing the product in order to determine if it really will sell. This situation prevails when wholesales and/or retailers will not commit orders but rather take a "wait and see" position. The risk is then left up to the publisher.

Sandra: Now you can better understand why most people follow the more traditional path of submitting a prospectus to an established publisher. After signing a contract, the author then submits the manuscript in return for a flat fee or a royalty on each copy sold.

Question: You've had your own business for five years and you've had many interesting and valuable experiences. What advice do you have for nurses who are highly motivated to start their own business?

Sandra and Chris: The process of starting up a new business has many common ingredients regardless of whether the new enterprise is service-oriented or manufacturing. Based upon our experience, here are a few suggestions:

1. During the period when you are getting really enthusiastic about starting your own business, spend some time determining what will be required to make this venture a success. Be realistic in your estimate of the time, money, and other resources that will be needed to start and sustain your business until it can support itself and you too. Plan carefully and the execution will be simplified.

2. You can greatly reduce your own personal financial risk if you can start your business without leaving your present job. If this procedure is not possible but your spouse can support the entire family, then you still have an advantage. Otherwise, be prepared to live off your savings until your business can support you.

3. If you believe in yourself and your ability to create something new, then be willing to take a risk. Your hard work and sacrifices will be rewarded many times over as you experience the freedom of "being your own boss."

4. Most entrepreneurs assume that the entire universe is eagerly awaiting their new service or product. Do not underestimate the time it takes to "get things done." Obtaining permits, opening bank accounts, and making other arrangements are time-consuming activities that do not generate revenue for you but must be done. Do not assume that the market will suddenly embrace you and your business. The marketplace is busily moving along under its own momentum. Many buyers are reluctant to try something new and even more prospects are unwilling to consider change.

5. Obtain expert professional advice and pay for it. It takes time and money to accomplish this process but effective advice can save

you more time, money, and frustration in the long run. Personal friends usually are the poorest of advisers because they (a) lack expertise, (b) get caught up in your euphoria, and (c) are reluctant to hurt your feelings or give you negative feedback. Outside advice is very helpful for all aspects of setting up your new business—office space and equipment, mailing regulations, letterhead design, and so on.

Two important areas of outside help are legal and accounting. The accounting function is essential to ascertain that you maintain proper records and file accurate and timely tax returns. Retain an attorney who specializes in small business and partnership law. Just because a neighbor or friend practices law, that does not mean that he or she has a good background in small business matters.

6. Be very wary of partnerships—many business partnerships are formed as a result of one unsure person talking a *more* unsure person into starting a business. The two then provide mutual support and reinforcement. Often, they fail to focus on the most important aspects of making the business successful.

If a partnership arrangement truly provides mutual advantage for you both, then you should draft a partnership agreement with advice from your attorney. This document should define your business, describe what each of you brings to the enterprise as well as your respective responsibilities and commitments, and, perish the thought, outline the mechanism for dissolving the partnership. The partnership agreement should be drafted and signed at an early stage in the partnership, when you both are enthusiastic, optimistic, and trusting. As circumstances change, you can modify your agreement if you agree on what should be changed. If you cannot agree, then your partnership is in trouble, and the sooner you know this, the better off you'll be in the long run.

A very important event for us was the dissolution of the original partnership business. We did not have a written agreement and the process of dissolution was very difficult and expensive. However, dissolving the original business allowed us the freedom to grow and develop in a way that would have been impossible due to differences in perspective and goals with the original partners. On balance, our advice would be to avoid partnerships but to use outside consultants and hire employees who are essential to meet your ongoing business needs.

7. Partnership versus incorporation—this is a complicated topic

because there are the usual financial, tax, and other factors to consider. We incorporated right away when we set up our own business. The corporation to us is a third party and we can deal with the corporation in terms of its restrictions, freedoms, and procedures without getting into the personal discussions that characterize a partnership. In addition, we have a third member on our board of directors who provides objectivity, fresh ideas, and reinforcement. We still control the organization and its operations, but having the corporate structure has helped us very much.

We hope our experiences will be helpful to other nurses who want to pursue an entrepreneurial enterprise.

5

Seminars on Sexuality (SOS)

Sharon Goldsmith
Rona Lee Cohen

Sharon's Story

Once upon a time in the small California town of Fullerton, a baby girl was born to a very special couple. The father of the baby was a minister, loved and respected, a pillar of the community. The mother of the baby was a lovely and dutiful wife.

As the girl grew, she watched her father's tireless efforts to bring peace, order, and meaning to the lives of his parishioners. She heard vivid tales of valor and self-sacrifice in distant mission fields. She knew her mother wanted to be a nurse.

By and by, it happened that the little girl became a young lady. No longer was she free to dream and play. No longer could she bask in the tender loving care of her family. The time had come to make a life for herself. She contemplated her choices. She investigated teaching. She considered becoming a stewardess. She dismissed secretarial work. Finally, she decided to be a nurse. Now she could be of service while she waited for the man of her dreams, and nursing would always come in handy if anything ever happened to him. She attended nursing school as was the custom, then graduate school, and in time met a handsome young doctor. They were married and of course she expected to live happily ever after.

This story has the perfect ending for a young woman growing up in the fifties. Career options were limited and obvious, the goal of marriage and family was primary, anatomy was destiny. Or was it? Even then, long before Betty Friedan lifted her pencil, I sensed a vague uncertainty within me. Perhaps it began when my high-school counselor suggested that I go to a university nursing program rather than to the hospital nursing program I had selected. "You have definite leadership potential," she assured me. Indeed, it appeared that I did. I went directly from a baccalaureate program at UCLA into a master's program at the same university, having worked all through undergraduate school on the university hospital wards as an aide by title but practically a team leader by responsibility. Although I had a good deal of exposure to capable floor nurses including head nurses and supervisors, my role models were always outstanding nursing instructors.

Upon graduation, I was immediately accepted as an instructor of nursing at California State University at Los Angeles and within two years was promoted to assistant professor. No question, I was on my way to an academic career. I just never took it seriously. I was biding my time until I could retire and have babies.

Soon after my promotion, my son was born, followed two years later by my daughter. For three and a half years I never for a moment questioned my role as wife and mother, nor do I regret for a moment those days now. However, when my son was nine months old, I became very active in La Leche League, an international non-profit organization that promotes breastfeeding through education and support. As expected, I soon became a group leader and, after a couple of years, professional liaison for Southern California and Nevada. Again, as with my earlier role models, it was the teaching function of the La Leche League leader that interested me.

I gave breastfeeding classes for women and couples in the West Los Angeles area for nearly seven years as my children grew, and periodically toyed with the idea of returning to the profession of nursing. Perhaps it no longer interested me. Perhaps I was insecure about my skills after so many years. Maybe it was a bit of both. Whatever the reason, I kept postponing my decision to return.

La Leche League itself (or perhaps its founding mothers) became an important mentor for me. Here was an organization developed by young mothers out of their kitchens—a "cottage shop" in its purest sense. These women were able to stir a pot on the stove with one hand, answer the phone for a breastfeeding counseling call with the other while stopping frequently to nurse a new infant or soothe an older child. This concept appealed to me very much—the ability to create a meaningful experience for people, fill an important informational void, and still be primarily a homebody.

The founding mothers had really accomplished something significant. They had collected all available information on breastfeeding, evaluated it, and reproduced what they found to be useful and effective. They selected a medical advisory board, they authored a book and a series of excellent pamphlets, they sent out a monthly newsletter, and within two years they expanded from a single group to groups throughout the United States and a few other countries. All groups were led by La Leche League trained and approved leaders, offered a series of four monthly breastfeeding classes, and provided telephone counseling for mothers, fathers, and professionals with questions, at no charge. The international office also offered a selection of books and unique breastfeeding and child-rearing products for purchase.

All in all, it was a wonderful concept, and I envied the women who masterminded it. One thing bothered me, however. As the leader of one of the largest and most affluent groups in the country, it upset me that the women and couples could get all that we offered—excellent classes and endless counseling at all hours—absolutely free. Somehow I felt devalued. Even childbirth classes charged a nominal fee. The goal of the organization was to make information available to all. Consequently, there were always fund raisers (like bake sales), mail solicitations, and much concern over money.

At the peak of my activity within the organization, something very interesting came to my attention. I noticed that although the topic was breastfeeding, the questions all too often turned to sex. Equally interesting was the fact that I, a nurse, did not know the answers, nor did my physician husband. Most of the people I worked with were highly educated, since West Los Angeles is a university community (UCLA), and affluent, since we are adjacent to Beverly Hills. It became clear to me that if we had questions and concerns about sex, this must be a universal problem. The solution was obvious—the first school for sex!

I began teaching women's classes while simultaneously taking every available local community sex course and reading the current literature. From the living rooms of these women, and with their help, Seminars On Sexuality evolved—a body of facts on all aspects of sexuality presented in a supportive environment that encouraged discussion and feedback. We had shared recipes and child-rearing techniques. It seemed a natural extension to share sexual "tips" as well. Sexual anatomy and physiology, religion, culture and sex, sexual options (masturbation, oral sex, fantasies, anal lovemaking), sexual health care (contraception, cancer detection, prevention of sexually transmitted diseases), even how to raise a "sexually healthy" child were all covered in the six weekly three-hour sessions. The women even left each class with a "homework" assignment designed to assist them in exploring and developing their sexuality. I charged a nominal fee. The word began to spread. I left La Leche League.

A business was obviously beginning to take shape, but unlike a wise entrepreneur, I did not evaluate the economic potential, identify the financing, and plan specific goals. I was open for an idea, and I found it. I was not concerned initially about profitability. I was interested in being of service. Most of the women who assisted me with administrative chores in those early days were of the volunteer mentality as well, since we all came from the same organization. Our big step, our risk so to speak, was to charge for our services. We charged $15 for a year of monthly sessions, and, miracle of miracles, a few women paid us even though they were used to getting information and support free from La Leche League. They continued to pay us when we changed the format to six weekly sessions and raised the price to $40. (The course costs $175 now.)

It was not long before staffing with volunteers caught up with me. I was determined to expand and found myself and a friend, who helped me write the original course, working long hours while our volunteer team worked sporadically when they felt like it. Print deadlines had to be met, recruitment phone calls had to be made, facilities had to be identified and reserved. My friend and I were doing it all. In order to handle the writing and administrative tasks, I decided to get someone who could help with teaching and recruitment. The first person I turned to was Rona Lee (Cookie) Cohen, a nurse whom I had met while participating in a research project on breastfeeding. The forces that brought her to this point are best described in her own words.

Cookie's Story

There were always two main interests in my family—medicine and music. My father was a dentist, my mother was a concert pianist, her mother was a nurse. I had always loved music and studied the piano since I was six, but it had nothing to do with science or with helping people. Medicine intrigued me more. Whenever someone in my family was hospitalized, I would be there, looking in every room, wanting to know what was wrong with the other patients.

It was clear that I would pursue a medical career. The question was, in what direction? Would it be dental hygiene, medicine, or nursing? To sort this out, I worked in my father's dental office for a few years during school vacations. I enjoyed being with my father's patients and caring for them, but by the time I was fifteen, I realized dentistry was too narrow a field for me. I considered becoming a doctor but hesitated for several reasons. It was the mid-fifties and I was afraid that I would be unable to combine marriage and family with medical training and practice. I also knew that few women were admitted to medical school, and I didn't want to fight that hard to "make it."

My parents, particularly my father, played a major role in my choosing nursing instead of medical school. They encouraged my brother to pursue a medical or dental career. (He is now a dentist.) They expected me to take up nursing. Although I decided not to enter medicine, my strongest role models have always been the women doctors I have worked with.

Deciding how and where to obtain my training was as crucial as my decision to become a nurse. I chose to go to a major university (Ohio State University) so I could earn my bachelor's degree while becoming a nurse. I felt this degree would give me a better chance for higher pay and leadership positions, which it did. It also paved the way for the nursing career I am now pursuing outside the traditional system.

The one thing I remember clearly from my schooling is that we were taught to apply the basic principles of nursing under any situation. From the day I graduated, I felt capable of taking on challenging positions. I was the only RN in a delivery room with no house physician, the sole recovery room nurse in a medium-sized hospital, a nurse in a Dutch-speaking hospital in Zwolle, Holland, knowing only ten words of Dutch.

I always saw nursing as hard work requiring difficult decisions, but perhaps the most frustrating thing about nursing for me was working in large institutions where change was so difficult to bring about. The politics of large hospitals and actual fear of trying something new bothered me no end. I felt that my ideas were years ahead of most of my nursing contemporaries. For example, when I implemented Family Centered Maternity Care at Cedars of Lebanon Hospital in Los Angeles, most of the nurses did not want the change and felt safer and happier with the old ways.

I saw so many of my colleagues follow in the same patterns day after day, not seeking, challenging, or questioning. Let someone else above take all the risks, was the attitude. If mistakes were made by doctors, a face-to-face confrontation was not attempted, only complaining behind their backs. I see myself as a risk taker, a challenger of old established patterns or rules, an aggressive individual who can get what I want while still being concerned about and sensitive to others. These traits made me ripe for the kind of opportunity SOS offered.

I was working as a Family Planning Nurse Practitioner at UCLA when Sharon approached me. Sexual counseling was very much a part of my practice, and I had taken special training in sexuality at UCLA. I began by teaching SOS women's classes and soon became a co-director of the organization.

The Team

Cookie and I joined forces. We had different but complementary characteristics. She was a better recruiter; I was a better writer. Whereas the approval of others has always been very important to me, Cookie thrives on being different. I prefer more structure; she chooses less. When I'm discouraged, she musters strength.

We possess important similarities too. We are both good teachers. We both love attention and yet are not threatened by each other's skills or charisma. Both of us are willing to take risks. We risk rejection every time we ask someone to take the class. We risk having no one show up every time we schedule a class or an event. We risk our reputations each time we go on radio or television, in fact each time we give a class, because our views about sex are not always popular. I am not certain though that anyone can be considered a real risk taker unless he or she has had to risk money, and up to this point, neither of us has been required to do that.

Recently, we added an associate director, Kay Coulson, to fill in the remaining gaps in our team. Kay, another RN, is a multitalented woman. She came to work for SOS from the administrative echelons of La Leche League, having been with us in spirit from the beginning. She contributes all the general office, bookkeeping, and administrative skills that Cookie and I lack.

The Seminars

It was not long after Cookie and I joined forces that women began requesting a similar SOS program for their partners. They stated that they would find them waiting up each night to hear what happened and ready to enthusiastically participate in the "homework." A couples program was developed in response to this request, with the format geared more toward sexual communication with a partner than toward self-exploration.

During this period, Seminars On Sexuality began to be recognized in the local community as an innovative and highly effective program. Referrals began to expand from simple word of mouth to professional recommendation. Cedars-Sinai Medical Center, Kaiser-Permanente Medical Centers, and the UCLA Human Sexuality Program began to request speeches and send clients, as did private psychotherapists and gynecologists. The therapists found that Seminars On Sexuality could facilitate the therapeutic process; the gynecologists found it could save them hours of counseling.

Our most recent development is an SOS program for teen girls, and it is perhaps the most exciting and promising of all. Adult graduates had been telling us for years they wished they had been through SOS when they were teenagers. A program for teen boys is scheduled next, with a men's program to follow. As of Fall, 1981, over 2500 people have taken one of the six-week SOS programs. An equal number have attended special one-session programs.

We offer sexuality classes for women, couples, and teen women in Los Angeles and the San Fernando Valley continuously throughout the year. The regularity has been very important, since the doctors and therapists who refer to us can always count on classes being available. We also function as a unique referral service for people who need gynecology, sex therapy, and general psychotherapy referrals. In October 1980 we were honored by Tom Bradley, the mayor of Los Angeles, and by the Los Angeles County Board of Supervisors for sponsoring National Family Sex Week in Los Angeles.

Building a Seminar Business

We have been conducting business officially from our office in Beverly Hills for the past two and a half years, and for five years before that from our kitchens. During the early years our growth came solely from word of mouth. Cookie and I knew many people in the West Los Angeles area. Her contacts were from several jobs and research projects. Mine came from years of working with breastfeeding women and couples. We both had numerous social contacts as well. Since we were highly respected as friends, colleagues, and teachers, people trusted us with a subject like sex and took our class. They were more than pleased when they had completed it and consequently told their friends.

Soon after we started, we were able to run a couple of classes every six weeks and break even. The question was, how long were we willing to just break even? If we were to become really profitable we needed to increase our prices and run more classes. We were both certain that we wanted to grow. The next question was how to increase our exposure. We knew word of mouth worked. How could we capitalize more on word of mouth—or should we invest in expensive advertising? We were beginning to develop a small but steady stream of referrals from physicians and psychotherapists. How could we increase our referral base? The questions were legion: the answers were few.

We developed graduate seminars to reinforce and support graduates. We carefully followed up on all prospective clients. We contacted professional colleagues. We managed to get some excellent television and radio exposure. It all helped and gradually boosted us from two adult groups per session to as many as four adult groups and one teen group per session. We were very excited and encouraged. The profit margin remained about the same, however, because our overhead suddenly increased. We rented an office as a base of operations and to handle all the books and equipment. We hired an associate director-administrator to handle all the day-to-day business, which by now was interfering with our home life. We upgraded all our printed materials (e.g., workbooks and brochures).

Throughout this period, we neglected to identify specific goals for profitability. We carefully set our goals for numbers of groups and numbers of individuals per group, and often came very close to meeting them. The numbers, however, were always based on breaking even. This occurred for several reasons. First, we were working so hard just to break even, we couldn't imagine adding to our recruitment load by increasing our goals. Second, we were just delighted to see people paying for what we enjoyed doing anyway. Finally, we kept thinking some breakthrough would occur that would catapult us to success. Indeed, what appeared to be that breakthrough did come along.

A friend of mine who owns a relatively new but extremely successful business happened to see me being interviewed on a local television show. He had watched SOS grow from its infancy and had periodically indicated an interest in becoming a financial backer if and when we were ready to expand. He called the morning after the screening to announce that he and his partner felt the time for expansion was right. Needless to say, Cookie, Kay, and I all jumped at this opportunity. SOS incorporated and its ownership went from two partners to four. Nirvana, it seemed, was just round the corner.

We immediately set the wheels of expansion in motion. We changed the location of the classes and introductory seminars from homes to public facilities to ensure respectability, simplify directions, and allow for increased numbers. Initially, we used temples and churches to keep costs down but finally had to switch almost entirely to hotels where services (e.g., coffee and room setup) were more reliable. We combined groups to increase the size, hoping to justify the room costs. We had to train and hire individuals as room managers to assist the group leader, since the size of each group and its organizational aspects were beyond one person's capacity. We added a highly paid marketing expert to our staff. We doubled the price of the class.

Now, instead of needing 50 people five times a year to break even, we needed 200 people five times a year just to break even. It seemed a bit overwhelming at first, but with a product as superb as ours, this amount of business seemed well within the range of probability, and everything beyond that magic figure of 200 people per session would be pure profit. It didn't work. With all the influx of money and ideas, and in spite of the new image, one year later recruitment seemed to be frozen at the old rate, perhaps even beginning to drop.

What happened? Was the seminar business simply not profitable, or was it just that our seminar had peaked? It is true that the seminar business is an extremely difficult one to make profitable unless the seminars are short in length and adaptable to very large groups (300 to 500 people per room), but we only needed to find 200 people per session in a city of three million. It also seemed unlikely that SOS had reached its peak. People seemed as excited about it as ever. Clearly, our errors lay elsewhere. We found them in marketing and sales. When our director of marketing took over, Cookie and I naturally pulled back from the area of direct sales. I began to explore literary and video opportunities; she began to focus on professional contacts like creating a conference with Children's Hospital of

Los Angeles on developmental sexuality for physicians and other
health professionals; he turned his attention to creating a corporate
image instead of beating the pavement. What should have been a
period of unprecedented growth was instead a setback.

Slowly, the options crystallized. Cut the overhead immediately by
eliminating the most costly item, the director of marketing. Resume
all previously effective recruitment techniques (speeches, telephone
follow-up, professional contacts, etc.), and vigorously pursue literary
and video opportunities.

Goals

Seeing our dreams shattered has been a sobering experience, but
there is a bright side too. We now have a clear immediate goal. To
build recruitment to 100 people per session five times per year or
about double our present rate. At that point, SOS will not only
break even but begin to show a margin of profit. To facilitate
profitability, we are exploring alternative office and classroom
facilities, since our rental bill eats up nearly one-third of our present
budget. We are also cutting another large expenditure, printing, by
increasing the volume of our print orders, thus greatly reducing the
cost per piece. We feel confident that a concerted effort to build
recruitment by conventional means accompanied by a commitment to
cut costs wherever possible will result in a business that is not only
notable but profitable.

Two other goals also run neck and neck with recruitment and in-
directly facilitate it. First, we plan to expand our sex education program to private schools. Los Angeles has recently experienced an incredible white flight from the public school system due to busing.
Each one of the new private schools, as well as each one of the old
established ones, faces the issue of how to provide sex education for
its burgeoning student body. One of the oldest and most respected
private schools in the city just contracted with SOS to provide its sex
education. The other schools will be likely to follow. Our other immediate goal, and perhaps the most exciting one, is to publish a
book on the history, evolution, and philosophy of SOS. A book will
not only facilitate recruitment, but will also expose many more people to accurate sex information than could ever be reached by classes
alone. This project as well as video possibilities are now being coordinated by our literary agent.

Finally, we have an ambitious goal for the future. We hope eventually to see an SOS center in every large city across the country.

These centers, like the one here in Los Angeles, would be reputable sources of sex information in their own communities, and in addition to offering services would strive to raise consciousness about responsible sexuality. Our media exposure and constantly growing group of graduates are accelerating our progress in this direction.

The Price

Developing this business has been fascinating and often very rewarding, but never easy. As nurses from traditional backgrounds, neither of us was prepared for the financial and administrative aspects of owning our own business. We have lost both money and clients through mistakes in selection of personnel. We have learned some painful lessons by trial and error, like which printers and graphics people we can count on, how many introductory seminars we need to fill a class, which facilities run smoothly, and so on. We have paid high fees for consultants and found it advisable to take on partners with financial and business expertise.

The cost of running our own business can be calculated in more than money. Our husbands and children have had to learn to be superbly patient, as business so often takes priority over family activities, or at least postpones them. When the business is yours, the job is done when it's finished, not just because the shift is over, and there is a tendency to feel you should always be working.

Cookie's family handles her commitment somewhat differently than mine does. Her parents (her father is now deceased) have always encouraged and supported her, while cautioning her to take time for her family. Her husband's parents feel that a woman belongs not in the business world but at home with her husband and children.

Her husband has given her financial assistance whenever necessary and in many ways is proud of what she has accomplished. However, having less of her time has been difficult for him. Her two boys, ages seventeen and eleven, would rather have her at home more. All in all, her strongest supporters have been her close friends as well as women within the SOS organization.

As for me, my greatest support has been from my husband. For the first twenty years I have known him, he has always encouraged me to do what I wanted or needed to do. His long-term compelling interest in the piano has also perhaps provided good modeling for my persistence. He has always willingly helped with the kids and the chores and never made me feel guilty for jobs undone. In fact, even now as I write this chapter, he is cooking a special Sunday breakfast for me. I think his most important contribution, however, has been his willingness to let me talk for hours on end about my problems, conflicts, and accomplishments, often taking priority over his equally important concerns. He has arranged speeches for me in the medical community, has frequently referred his own patients, and has encouraged his colleagues to do the same.

My children, ages thirteen and eleven, have had a bit more difficulty with my career. It has affected them in two ways. First, it is a difficult one to explain to their friends, and since I am frequently on radio and television, they are questioned. "My mother teaches sex" is often greeted with mixed responses. Their close friends, however, seem to have no problem with this, and in fact enjoy their access to good sex education materials. My daughter's sixth-grade teacher commented to her recently that she had seen me on a very popular evening magazine show. Needless to say, my daughter had mixed feelings.

Second, they have watched me leave at least one evening a week and frequently two or three and work during many of the hours they are home, so I'll get comments like, "You're not going out again?" or "Don't you ever stay home?" I try to make it up by always seeing them off in the morning and spending time alone with each of them in the evening as often as possible.

My parents live locally and therefore, like my children, must "explain me" to their friends and parishioners. Although my father has difficulty with the type of work I do, he understands the need from his own counseling. My mother is not only uncomfortable with what I do, but also questions my reasons for working when I don't have to. She has also suggested that someday I may regret spending so much time away from my family.

Both Cookie and I feel that the stress level in our lives is relatively high. We often bring the problems of the day home with us and find them affecting our family life. SOS is a people business and brings with it all the associated problems—finding good people, supporting them, boosting productivity, and the like. It also has all the problems that come from relying on suppliers (printers, hotels, the Post Office, etc.). Finally, since it is viewed by many as a luxury, SOS business fluctuates with the economy perhaps more than most businesses. An optimum business for us would not be one without problems but one without recruitment problems. Of course, the only way to make that happen is to be certain we are out there selling.

Success won't just happen; we have to make it happen!

The Rewards

It is important to end this chapter with a clear idea of the rewards of an undertaking like SOS. First of all, both Cookie and I can say that it is a business that is full of surprises. There is no such thing as a dull business day. There is always a piece of mail, a phone call, or a visit from someone we didn't expect.

Second, although any job has responsibilities, being your own boss allows you to arrange your time to your advantage. If shopping and lunch are on the agenda, work can usually be switched to evening hours. We have potentially more flexibility to meet our families' needs than if we were tied up in one place nine hours a day plus travel time.

Next, there have been many positive effects on our families and on our personal lives. As working women and particularly entrepreneurial women, we have come to appreciate in a very personal way the worries, stresses, and indeed the successes of our husbands, whereas before we both underestimated their concerns and took their success for granted. Our children of necessity have learned to be more independent and self-sufficient, skills that will serve them well as adults. Our busy lives have also serviced us in another way. Because of tight schedules, we must practice what SOS "preaches" which is to take "Prime Protected Time" with one's partner on a regular basis.

We have learned to reduce the effects of stress by watching our nutrition and rest, and both of us have maintained a vigorous exercise program for several years now. Because of this, we both look better physically at age forty than at any other time in our lives.

The last, and perhaps the most important, reward for both of us is the way we affect the lives of the men, women, and children we touch. Each time we give a piece of vital information, clarify a situation, or provide an option that didn't exist, we are rewarded. Each time we watch an individual improve the quality of his or her life, we are inspired to accept the challenge to continue our efforts to provide this unique educational program.

The greatest obstacle to our success has not been skill, prescribed roles, family obligations, stress, or money. Closed minds and frozen viewpoints will always be our most formidable foes. In spite of the sexual revolution, or perhaps because of it, many people remain uncomfortable with sex and avoid confronting the issues for themselves and for their children. To make sex education a legitimate concern for all is an enormous goal, but if we can even begin to reach it, future generations will be able to achieve a natural balance between sex and other aspects of life. There can be no greater prize.

We would certainly encourage more women in nursing to enter the business world either as private practitioners or in some phase of nursing and business that is totally innovative like SOS. The marriage of nursing and business presents multiple challenges and requires many skills but offers the flexibility, control, and satisfaction often unavailable in an institutional setting. It is a wonderful feeling to be able to say, "It's mine!"

6

Perinatal Dimensions:
A Successful Beginning

Patricia A. Allen
Dorothy B. Turner

Perinatal Dimensions is a young firm, still becoming established after two years of development. During that time we have experienced some ups and downs, and in the process we have grown and learned a number of points about developing a successful business. This chapter is written with the intent of being useful to other nurses contemplating or jumping into the exciting arena of business. It traces the evolution of Perinatal Dimensions, highlighting the process of our resocialization from nurses to businesswomen.

Planning and Development

After two years of developing a nursing firm, we think of Perinatal Dimensions as successful and regard that mind-set as essential. Feeling successful generates the energy to continue despite the obstacles that arise from time to time. The availability of energy, in turn, is a key factor in creative thinking and planning.

Webster's (1961) defines success as "a favorable termination of a venture; often, specifically the attainment of wealth, favor, or eminence." This definition speaks to gaining dollars, position, status, or fame, and to the outcome of a venture. In addition, we think that success can be measured according to goals attained, standards of quality met, skills refined, and personal and professional growth. Therefore, process success as well as outcome success can be assessed. Both are important to the vitality of a business venture.

Early in the development of Perinatal Dimensions we learned that successful process does not guarantee successful outcome. Nevertheless, we enjoyed the process success and realized it could lead to an outcome success at the time and place in question or at another time and place. For example, we once approached a shared services group of small community hospitals, proposing a group purchase of a neonatal educational program. The group decided not to purchase the program, because members stated that the volume of deliveries in the hospitals was too low to justify the expenditure. We analyzed the steps in the negotiation process, the written proposal, and the marketing plan. We were convinced that the concept was sound and the proposal well developed. Our negotiation skills had improved markedly and we had tried a new marketing approach. Although we did not have a successful financial outcome, we experienced a process success.

Background Perspective

For a decade each of us worked within several systems and in a variety of professional nursing positions to participate in the evolution of regionalized perinatal care in Ohio. We have known the pain and frustration of admitting a severely asphyxiated infant to the intensive care nursery via transport from the region while realizing this tragic event is largely preventable. Yet, in the same week at a conference we listened to nurses from community hospitals expressing a sincere commitment to high-quality care. We recognized that a key factor for improved pregnancy outcome is an effective mechanism for continuing education so that personnel in all centers are skilled in the early identification of perinatal problems, resuscitation and stabilization of infants, and appropriate referrals of high-risk mothers and infants. As members of a perinatal team we have been acutely aware that the demands of operating an intensive care unit and simultaneously conducting an outreach education program are overwhelming. Such problems as insufficient number of personnel, inadequate budgets, uncertain funding status, and multiple needs of constituent hospitals have been cited repeatedly by perinatal educators across the country.

The need for an effective mechanism for continuing education coupled with uncertain prospects for meeting the need propelled us into exploring new approaches. Concurrently, we were fatigued by the prevailing stressors of the tertiary center and ready for a change. We contemplated the issue of community responsibility for continuing education and wondered if community hospitals would make a financial investment to support perinatal continuing education programs in their facilities. If hospitals did invest in continuing education, would the probability of improved care practices be increased? We began to explore the idea of designing a continuing education service that would be directed to the community hospital and offered as a fee-for-service model.

Over a period of several weeks we brainstormed about educational topics to be developed and the prospective market for them. We debated the marketing advantages and disadvantages of specializing in perinatal education only, or broadening into pediatric clinical topics, or perhaps into behavioral and management areas. We discussed a range of services that might be offered, including education programs, clinical nursing services, clinical program development, and consultation.

While solidifying ideas about the services we would offer and the model for continuing education, we consulted with colleagues at tertiary centers, the state health department, schools of nursing, and professional organizations, as well as with community leaders in voluntary health organizations.

Generally the reaction was this: "We think it is needed; we think your approach is sound; we don't know anyone doing it and we don't know if it will work, but we encourage you to try it."

From site visits to community hospitals, participation in professional organizations and workshops, and informal discussions with community hospital personnel, we had recognized an interest in updating their knowledge and skills in perinatal care. We also acknowledged the financial risks involved in testing an innovative approach in an undeveloped market. However, we were confident about the need, about our ability to produce a quality program, and about our willingness to take risks and accept challenge. Therefore, we decided to offer a range of services to include education, consultation, and program development specific to perinatology. Services would be selected carefully to avoid overextending ourselves and lessening the quality of our offerings, as well as to limit production cost, particularly at the beginning. Developing the educational services for community hospitals would be the first phase of operation, expanding when feasible into consultation and program development at community hospitals. The next phase of operation would be the development of similar services for centers offering complex perinatal services.

Design of the Educational Service

A regionalized system of perinatal health services has evolved in Ohio, as in the United States, over the past two decades. Tertiary centers have been developed to address the complex problems of sick infants. Specialized personnel from several disciplines and rapidly advancing knowledge and technology have come together to reduce the neonatal mortality and morbidity and to support the families of high-risk infants. Most infants are delivered in community hospitals. Their survival and the quality of the survivorship are influenced significantly by the knowledge and skills of personnel who provide care during the perinatal period.

As advances in perinatal care were made, it became apparent that improvement in care practices in community hospitals progressed at a slower rate than at regional centers. Problems such as those identified by Kattwinkel and associates (1978) interfere with effective delivery of perinatal care and negatively influence the outcomes of pregnancy on communities:

1. Inadequate equipment and inadequate knowledge regarding use of basic equipment
2. Inadequate or absent hospital policies for identification and treatment of high-risk infants and mothers
3. Inadequate knowledge of basic perinatal care principles
4. Nonfacilitating attitudes toward perinatal care leading to a tendency of nonintervention prior to, or even after, identifying pathology

Because of such problems, the concept of outreach perinatal education has evolved. A number of methods have been used, such as regional workshops, one-day workshops on site, and mini-residencies at regional centers. Educational efforts using these traditional educational methods have been met with some resistance because of factors relating directly to the educational methods and to attitudes of community hospital personnel. Maisels and associates (1978), Kattwinkel (1978), and others have concluded that traditional methods of education do not have optimal effects in changing care practices. The following deficiencies have been identified regarding educational methods:

1. The educational exposure is superficial, because of limited time and subject presentation.
2. The material presented often is oriented to practice in the intensive care setting rather than the community hospital and therefore is not utilized in the community hospital.
3. The population reached often is only one group of professionals (usually nurses), therefore enhancing already existing barriers of communication and acting as a deterrent to progressive change.

Our goals were to offer a specialized, high-quality educational service that would be relevant to the community hospital setting and to assist personnel in translating current knowledge into practice. We were impressed with the concepts and accomplishments of the University of Virginia program (Kattwinkel et al. 1979) and decided to incorporate several of its features into the Perinatal Dimensions model. The design of our educational service is built on a consultation model. The approach involves active participation by community personnel and is individualized to the educational needs and goals of the community hospital. Features of the service are as follows:

1. Hospital self-assessment
   a. Employs self-assessment tools to enable hospital staff to identify goals and actual capabilities
   b. Involves active participation by hospital staff
2. Community-based program
   a. Implemented in the community hospital
   b. Oriented to practice in the community hospital
   c. Focused on the realities of day-to-day operations
3. Concentrated educational modules
   a. Present comprehensive, in-depth units of study
   b. Include theory and skills
   c. Designed to individualize instruction to hospital needs
4. Coordinated team approach
   a. Delivers presentations by physician-nurse team to physicians, nurses, and support personnel
   b. Enhances nurse-physician communication
   c. Increases uniformity of care practices

5. Cost-effectiveness
   a. Minimizes off-duty time
   b. Reduces staff travel expenses
   c. Yields high cost-benefit ratio

Educational topics offered in the phase one educational service to the community are listed in Table 6-1.

After several months of experience with this educational approach and the basic series of topics, we expanded the educational offerings to include current issues in perinatology and topics related to perinatal health services; we also added to the clinical series.

After working with larger hospital client systems that offered more complex services to perinatal patients, we further expanded the educational offerings to include leadership and effective communication development. In addition we began to market consultation and program-development services. These were:

1. Consultation
   a. Assessment of hospital perinatal services:
      Employs self-assessment tools, reviews, procedures, policies, medical records
      Interviews leadership personnel
      Summarizes findings in written report with recommendations
   b. Ongoing consultation:
      Identifies approaches for implementing planned organizational change
2. Program Development
   a. Curriculum design for orientation and other educational programs
   b. Development of standards, policies, and procedures
   c. Development of plan for recruitment and retention of personnel
   d. Development of plan for budgeting, scheduling, and utilization of personnel
   e. Development of clinical programs, e.g., family-centered services, parent education, follow-up care
3. Education
   a. Principles and practices of perinatal care includes physiological and psychosocial topics
   b. Current issues in perinatology, such as ethical dilemmas, coping with stress, primary nursing, nurse's attachments and grief

    c. Development of leadership and communication skills, for
       example: developmental tasks of leaders, decision making,
       assertiveness, team building.

Establishing the Firm

Parallel to the design and development of the services of Perinatal
Dimensions was the process of establishing the firm itself and
developing a marketing program.

After reviewing some "how to" literature about developing a
small business and consulting with experts in business and marketing,
we secured the services of an attorney and built the structure for the
firm. Selection of the name for the firm required lengthy deliberation. Several choices were identified, tested with colleagues and
friends for reactions, and rejected before choosing Perinatal Dimensions. A specialty name was selected to pinpoint the nature of the
services, and our attorney registered the name in the state of Ohio.

After reviewing the characteristics of a corporation and a partnership with our attorney, we decided to start with an equal partnership
with individual insurance coverage for professional liability. We
postponed the establishment of a corporation until assets would be
sufficient to need protection and corporate professional liability
coverage was required (i.e., when teaching involved hands-on
demonstrations with patients or advanced technical procedures).

We obtained an IRS employer number and established procedures
for taxes, salary and benefits, and budgeting. A simple accounting
system with a ledger of debits and credits was initiated and banking
relationships established. Although we were aware from the literature
that undercapitalization is a major factor in small business failure,
we decided that a small investment made by each of us would be sufficient to get started. Since our services were to be provided on site
to the client, we did not establish a separate office location and
decided instead to operate from one partner's home address with a
telephone answering service during business hours. No purchases of
capital equipment were required. We prepared a budget for each project undertaken as well as an overall budget for production and
operating expenses. Most of the early expenses were printing costs,
office supplies, long-distance telephone calls, and travel.

The Marketing Program

Early in our development we wrestled with the question: How do we market our services? Like many professionals, we equated marketing with selling; we did not wish to portray the image of "hard sell." Our goal was to offer a high-quality service for a reasonable cost.

Only recently have concepts of marketing been applied consciously in the delivery of professional services. Professionals are gaining awareness of the utility of an effective marketing program for the cost-effective delivery of services, achieving a more accurate match of services to the target population. In the field of perinatology, a number of major conferences have included presentations on marketing perinatal health services.

Analyzing the market for perinatal continuing education services was the first task in developing a marketing program for Perinatal Dimensions. The total market was divided into potential segments according to the following characteristics:

1. Availability and accessibility of educational programs currently offered
2. Availability of resource personnel for continuing education
3. Availability of hospital financial support for continuing education
4. Availability of medical and nursing specialists
5. Demographic characteristics of the population served by the hospital
6. Perinatal services provided
7. Financial position of the hospital and the perinatal service
8. Geographic proximity

To quote Lovelock (1977):

> The concept of market segmentation is based upon the proposition that (1) consumers (hospitals) are different; (2) differences in consumers (hospitals) are related to differences in market behaviors; (3) segments of consumers (hospitals) can be isolated within the overall market.

Applying the concept of market segmentation facilitates analysis of the market and enhances the probability of success matching services and the needs and desires of the market (Fryzel 1978).

The market segment we selected was the community hospital having the following characteristics:

1. Located within 150 miles from current continuing education offerings

2. Limited numbers of continuing education resource personnel
3. Financial support for one or two staff members to attend continuing education offerings
4. Limited number of perinatal specialists
5. 500-2500 deliveries per year
6. Services for healthy mothers and infants; stabilization and transport of high-risk population
7. Variable financial positions with respect to income from maternity unit
8. Located in central and southeastern Ohio

Marketing our Services

We accepted Kotler and Conner's (1977) definition of professional services marketing and built our marketing program on strategies they identified to produce disciplined growth:

> Professional services marketing consists of organized activities and programs by professional services firms that are designed to retain present clients and attract new clients by sensing, serving, and satisfying their needs through delivery of appropriate services on a paid basis in a manner consistent with creditable professional goals and norms.

The strategies, which we'll discuss in the following sections, are:

1. Service and market specialization
   Favorable awareness program
3. Identifying and cultivating high-potential prospective clients

Service and Market Specialization. The marketing literature indicates that one of the marketing errors professional firms make is to strike out in many directions for possible new clients and to develop a "total service" philosophy, which is counterproductive. Kotler and Conner identify two distinct advantages of specialization:

1. Specialization gives the firm a preferred position placing it automatically in contention for potential clients seeking that kind of expertise.
2. Specialization permits a greater profit on volume because the firm develops 'cutting edge' expertise and low cost procedures for handling recurrent situations. [Kotler and Conner 1977]

Table 6.1 Educational Topics

Module	Content	Skills
1. Identification of the high-risk mother	High-risk factors of pregnancy Evaluating fetal maturity and well-being	Internal and external monitoring
2. Immediate newborn assessment	Identification of the newborn at risk Significance of gestational age	Physical assessment of the newborn Dubowitz assessment
3. Resuscitation of the newborn	Identification of the newborn requiring resuscitation Techniques of resuscitation	Apgar scoring/Bag and mask ventilation Endotracheal intubation Cardiac massage Administration of medications
4. Thermoregulation	Principles of thermoregulation	Operating radiant warmer Operating isolette
5. Stabilization: respiratory system	Identification of respiratory distress Significance of blood gases Care of the infant with repiratory distress	Assessment of the respiratory system Umbilical artery catheterization Arterial blood sampling [a] Suctioning/Administration of oxygen
6. Stabilization: cardiovascular system	Transition from fetal to newborn circulation Fluid requirements of the sick newborn	Assessment of the cardiovascular system Measurement of blood pressure Starting peripheral intravenous fluids Dextrostix
7. Hyperbilirubinemia	Identification and care of the infant with hyperbilirubinemia	Phototherapy
8. The newborn with sepsis	Identification of the infected newborn Care of the infant with sepsis	Obtaining gastric aspirate Assisting with lumbar puncture Obtaining specimens for culture
9. Convalescent care of the growing premature infant	Environment promoting growth and development Nutritional needs for growth Monitoring apnea Preparation for homegoing: teaching parents	Weaning from isolette Techniques for infant stimulation Nasogastric feeding Placement of monitor leads Recording apneic episodes
10. Family-centered approach to care	Concept of family/Crisis intervention Attachment at risk/Perinatal loss and grief	Communication techniques

a Neonatalogist will assist in teaching these skills.

We chose a specialty-linked name for the firm and therefore began
to concentrate on specialty services. Within the specialty our interests
included a range of consultation and education services to a wide
market of community and tertiary centers; however, we decided to
build one service at a time for a specific market segment and to
develop it well before expanding to another. The brochure introducing the services of Perinatal Dimensions describes the specialized
package for continuing education and is directed to the community
hospital. It lists other services available, but the thrust is specific to
continuing education.

Favorable Awareness Program.   The goals we developed for
gaining favorable awareness were to create market visibility, establish
credibility, and build a reputation. We wished to portray Perinatal
Dimensions as specialized, of high quality, competent, reliable, innovative, and client-centered. Specific activities to build favorable
awareness included these:

1. Designing a logo
2. Selecting stationery and business cards
3. Developing a brochure describing services
4. Offering a conference by means of a national mailing list
5. Attending professional meetings
6. Public speaking in the community
7. Obtaining a personalized telephone answering service

Design of the logo and printed materials involved working closely
with an artist. We rejected the symbolism of storks, rattles, and
mothers with babies; instead we emphasized the firm's name, working to achieve simplicity, dignity, and visual impact. Reviewing the
materials of several companies, we noted that successful firms made
effective use of texture, color, and design to enhance the corporate
image.

Offering a conference with national mailing of the brochure, attending professional meetings, and public speaking in the community
were important activities in our becoming established in the professional community as a private firm, since we were known previously
in the context of positions held in systems.

The telephone is an effective business tool in conveying an initial
impression. Because a full-time secretary was not in the budget, we
considered the advantages and disadvantages of an answering service
versus a mechanical device for recorded messages. We chose the

answering service because it offered several advantages: a person answering with the firm's name; an opportunity to interact with the telephone secretary; service during regular business hours; reasonable cost. Initially we discussed the nature of our business with the telephone secretary and later received feedback from clients that was courteous and reliable.

Identifying and Cultivating High-Potential Prospective Clients. Kotler and Conner listed criteria for favorable prospective clients, which included high growth and profit potential, actual or potential dissatisfaction with their current firm, a base for attracting further clients in that industry, and the availability of a good contact or referral source. We have identified the following steps for developing new clients:

1. Generating and evaluating prospective clients from personal referrals and other contacts
2. Initiating contact with the prospective client through an individualized, personalized approach of telephone, then sending a follow-up letter and brochure
3. Entry into the client's system for a meeting to discuss the services of Perinatal Dimensions; projecting the firm as client-centered and free from institutional bias or licensure clout
4. Presenting a proposal with services and costs

Early responses to our marketing strategies have been encouraging. Several clients have been engaged, and others have expressed interest in the services of Perinatal Dimensions. We have learned that smaller community hospitals are less likely to purchase the services than are those with a delivery service of 1200 per year or more, or those planning or offering services to high-risk mothers and infants.

A barrier we had not anticipated fully was the apparent threat our firm poses in terms of being perceived as influencing patient referral patterns. This perceived threat resulted in efforts to block our entry into several hospitals. Those actions created an additional challenge to the marketing of our continuing education services; however, as the firm moved into the expanded services of consultation and program development that barrier diminished.

Pricing

Our goal in determining pricing was to offer high-quality services for a reasonable cost. The questions were many: What was a reasonable cost? What were the services worth in an undeveloped market? What were the psychic costs associated with changing established behavior patterns? Would hospitals purchase services from a new firm?

While holding earlier leadership positions, we had become comfortable discussing budgets, negotiating salaries, and accepting honoraria for professional presentations; however, we experienced some feelings of uncertainty and anxiety in establishing and presenting the fee schedule for the services of Perinatal Dimensions. We attempted to analyze our uneasiness about pricing and were able to pinpoint two bothersome issues: First, we were fully and individually responsible and accountable for the finances of our firm. The financial risks seemed real and frightening. Second, the worth of our services on the market was unknown. The situation required making our best estimate for pricing and then trying it. Pricing was a complex issue: to price too low might infer that the services were less than the high quality we planned to offer; to price too high would result in the services not being purchased.

We could find no established precedents for fee-for-service continuing education. Therefore we considered factors such as these: customary fees for workshops in the community; our production and marketing costs; cost containment constraints upon hospital budgets. We anticipated that clients would perceive a risk in purchasing an innovative service being offered by a new firm to an undeveloped market.

The Resocialization Process

A major discovery we made while presenting ourselves as representatives of a new business was the significant resocialization process that we required. We were comfortable with various roles in nursing, having had experience as teachers, clinicians, and consultants, so we were comfortable with the functions required to deliver the services of Perinatal Dimensions. We remembered previous role transitions from student to staff nurse to clinical nurse specialist and recalled a period of anxiety and uncertainty experienced with each step until the new status became known and comfortable. To enhance the taking on of the new role of nurse-businesswoman, we bombarded ourselves with a variety of readings from business and women's literature. This process not only helped us to conceptualize the new role but also increased our understanding of the business world. We became increasingly aware of the assets we possessed as nursing leaders that would enhance our success in the new business role. A major task in the resocialization process was to transpose those behavioral assets from the familiar context of nursing to the new and unfamiliar context of business. Accomplishing this task required thinking, acting, and looking successful.

Success: Thinking It

Positive mind-set is a crucial variable in creating a successful business. A conscious attitude of "as you think it, so it is" contributes to a sense of personal power and self-esteem in the new role. Thinking and acting positively yield positive results. We ascribe to this philosophy and therefore endeavored to build and reinforce a positive, confident mind-set about the firm. To do this we used strategies such as these:

1. Perceiving our firm as the primary career, contributing full-time energies and commitment to Perinatal Dimensions; viewing the part-time positions that supplemented our income as secondary positions
2. Listing reasons why the firm would succeed
3. Verbally picturing ourselves as successful businesswomen in various business encounters, thereby improving our ability to identify behaviors that needed to be added, deleted, or refined; working to develop selected behaviors in a safe environment.
4. Reinforcing the positive beliefs by praising each other's effective businesswoman behaviors; analyzing each business situation by criticizing each other's performance, praising new skills and effective behaviors; conquering fears of failure through this self-evaluation technique.
5. Producing carefully prepared written documents and high-quality programs; acknowledging our growing sense of accomplishment when positive feedback was received from recipients of our services
6. Maintaining a sense of humor and injecting fun into the changes we were making; enjoying clippings, mottos, spontaneous expressions of humor; being able to laugh at ourselves
7. Taking time for rest and self-renewal, including activities such as running, tennis, and walks in the woods.

Success: Acting It

As nurses we came to the business table with behavioral assets that we underestimated initially. Nursing roles had provided opportunities for listening, clarifying, reflecting, supporting, and directing in therapeutic relationships. While holding nursing positions we had achieved a high level of interpersonal competence. Interpersonal competence is the

> skill or set of abilities allowing an individual to shape the response he gets from others. This involves predicting the impact of one's own actions on the other person's definition of the situation, having a varied and large repertoire of possible lines of action and necessary interpersonal resources to employ appropriate tactics. . . experience, maturity, adaptability, openness and self-confidence will contribute to increased competence. [Fagin 1979]

Although we needed to refine negotiation skills and assertive responses in the business context, the interpersonal competence previously acquired was an asset in the strategic planning necessary for marketing and presenting the services of Perinatal Dimensions.

In addition to increasing our repertoire of interpersonal responses, we effected subtle changes in our speech and writing patterns that enhanced our business image. In the resocialization process we became increasingly aware of the nursing jargon we used habitually. Then we attempted to delete those terms and replace them with clear, direct language that would be understood by nonnursing health care professionals.

When making presentations of our services we used words that were meaningful to the audience. We listened carefully for key words and phrases that others, particularly administrators, used to interpret our services and later adopted some of them. As we gained self-confidence in the business role, we answered specific questions immediately and clarified points with self-assurance. Initially we hesitated at times with answers to questions regarding our services and fees. Although the hesitancy reflected our inexperience and anxiety in the business context, it might have been interpreted as uncertainty about providing the services.

In business meetings we were conscious also of our nonverbal behaviors. We aimed for a calm, rational, logical, confident manner, establishing direct eye-to-eye contact with the prospective client, speaking with a strong, confident voice, and expressing self-assurance by a professional yet relaxed body position conveyed the desired impression.

Success: Dressing It

Another conscious change in our self-presentation was dress. At first we scoffed at the notion presented by Molloy and others that choice of dress influences success in business, but as we observed successful men and women we realized that dress does seem to affect responses from people (Molloy 1977). Thereafter we chose clothing and accessories thoughtfully in order to obtain favorable responses. We selected traditional tailored lines and conservative colors. Simultaneously we blended our own personal tastes and individuality to create a successful look that also reflected each of our personalities. We rejected ruffles, frills, and flowered dresses as well as masculine-looking pantsuits. Generally our attire consisted of suits of jacket and skirt and blouse with bow or scarf, plain shoes, and leather attache case.

Renegotiation of Relationships

In former positions we had developed collegial relationships within systems and professional organizations. We did not anticipate the impact our assuming the business role would have on established professional relationships. There was uncertainty about what the appropriate behaviors were in the new relationship.

We raised some questions such as these regarding continuation of leadership positions within professional organizations: Did these positions involve a conflict of interest? Would we be perceived as using the organization forum to promote our business? These questions have not been answered fully in our minds. Some relationships will require further clarification over time. Also as professional nursing firms become more prevalent, patterns of relationships will become established and expectations will be clearer.

Summary and Future Directions

This chapter has traced the evolution of Perinatal Dimensions, a nursing firm for consultation, education, and program development in perinatal nursing. Future directions are under consideration and include continuing to develop a market for fee-for-service perinatal continuing education; expanding the services to include the development of broader topics or additional types of services; and testing the business behaviors while holding nursing leadership positions within a system.

References

Fagin, Claire M. "Refocus on Leadership." *Nursing Leadership* 2(4):6-13, December 1979.

Fryzel, Ronald. "Marketing Nonprofit Institutions." *Hospital and Health Services Administration* 23(1): 8-16, Winter 1978.

Kattwinkel, John; Cook, Lynn J.; Nowacek, George A.; Ivey, Hallam H.; and Short, Jerry G. "Improved Perinatal Knowledge and Care in the Community Hospital Through a Program of Self-Instruction." *Pediatrics* 64(4):451-458, October 1979.

Kattwinkel, John; Cook, Lynn J.; Nowacek, George A.; Short, Jerry G.; and Ivey, Hallam H. "Attitudes Toward Perinatal Care in Community Hospitals." *Pediatric Research* 12(4) part 2:446, April 1978.

Kotler, Phillip, and Conner, Richard A. "Marketing Professional Services." Journal of Marketing 41:71-76, January 1977.

Lovelock, Christopher. "Concepts and Strategies for Health Marketers." *Hospital and Health Services Administration* 22(4):50-62, Fall 1977.

Maisels, M. J.; Morrow, D.; Fernsler, S.; Hildebrandt, R. J. "Care of Low Birthweight and Sick Newborn Infants in Community Hospitals—Effect of an Education Program." *Pediatric Research* 12(4) part 2:446, April 1978,

Molloy, John T. *The Woman's Dress for Success Book*. New York: Warner Books, 1977.

Webster's New Collegiate Dictionary. Springfield, Mass: G. & C. Merriam, 1961.

7

Consulting and Workers' Compensation

Katharine Borges Thompson

For the last three years, I have functioned in the role of consultant in stress and pain management. The route I took to arrive at this point was not, needless to say, the shortest distance between two points. I will review how I happened to select this direction for my nursing practice and the new skills I learned in order to make the transition. Although the opportunity to change directions was partly an accident and luck, it took determination and willingness to take risks; much of my motivation to move into private practice came from my growing frustration with the usual job choices I found available to nurses, particularly those in bureaucratic systems.

The Buildup

I should have sensed that I would experience much disillusionment and disappointment in nursing as far back as 1963, when I taught in a diploma school of nursing. My brother, a recent high-school graduate, earned a larger salary than I. His job required no special training.

That experience was just the beginning of a fourteen-year period gaining skills in implementing change and learning how to advance the nursing profession, primarily in the hospital. Although I seemed successful in my work, I rarely saw lasting beneficial change; the nursing profession did not seem to be advancing, particularly at the staff nurse level, except in salaries.

While working in hospitals, I developed managerial skills and became quite adept at "putting out fires." Handling crises rather than planning and implementing long-range goals became my usual activity. Over time, I was increasingly distressed to see good ideas tabled and qualified, creative nurses becoming disenchanted. Except for a few instances, I felt as if I was continually starting over. For example, in one hospital, my job title and responsibilities changed three times in two years because of department reorganization. I have seen extremely gifted head nurses leave hospitals because of the drain that problems outside their control cause in interfering with quality care and development of staff nurses.

I don't mean to make the picture all bad. Instances of positive change have occurred, particularly outside hospitals. More often than not, however, qualified nurses are not able to achieve their potential. The systems where nurses are employed are part of the problem. In my opinion, though, we are a major cause of our own frustrations.

As a primarily female profession with a history of functioning in a subordinate role, we tend to see ourselves as less than other professions. I found myself struggling with my identity as a nurse. Many nurses measured their own competence against the medical profession rather than against nursing role models. Frequently nurses held in high esteem are the ones able to carry out medical procedures. When asked, many nurses find approval from physicians more significant than approval from nursing peers. I have experienced and seen bright nurses being complimented for their intelligence and then told "you should have been a doctor." Even other nurses have made such comments. I have experienced constant pressure to prove myself to other nurses while employed in the hospital system. I have noticed that nurses often do not hold peers in high esteem. This response is particularly an issue in solving problems or improving patient care. We have great difficulty following nursing orders. Instead, nurses report to one another, each carrying out nursing interventions as s/he prefers within the limits of policy and the physicians's orders. I think nurses carry democracy a bit too far. It was very interesting to me to go back into hospitals while following my own patients. Some nurses followed "suggestions" I offered; others saw me as an intruder. The difference was proving myself by getting to know the staff and participating in patient care conferences. What a shame that we have to go through so much to be accepted and listened to by other nurses.

Another issue that goes hand in hand with the above is accountability. I have noticed over the years that we tend to blame the system we're in—the doctors, nursing administration, and so forth—rather than take responsibility. This problem surfaces in patient care, nursing orders, and change making. I have seen nurses fearful of taking risks in both hospital and educational systems. To be identified outside the safety of the group is very difficult. I do not feel we are adequately socialized to function independently. I went through much uncertainty progressing in the areas of accountability and risk taking.

Before I left the hospital employment, I also learned about the business realities of providing health care. I was totally unprepared to deal with middle-management responsibilities, and learned on the job. It was painful to learn that wanting to give good care and being qualified to do so were not enough. I must give credit to my experience in hospitals for learning how to deal with such things as budgets and staffing, and confronting the reality that it costs money to provide care. Even that experience did not prepare me for being on my own. Whether in a hospital or educational system, my risk taking and efforts at independence were within a structured environment.

I left hospital nursing and reentered nursing education. Although I found it stimulating and enjoyed the students, I soon realized that I no longer wanted to provide care through others on a full-time basis. I wanted direct patient contact outside the hospital, clinic, or educational systems. Pressured by frustration and dissatisfaction, I looked for a different alternative.

The Search

I was reluctant to move immediately to independent practice for several reasons. First, I was insecure about generating an income. It was unlikely that I would qualify for insurance reimbursement for my services. I was not confident that I could build a practice of self-paying clients. Second, I was uncomfortable practicing private psychotherapy without clarification of the legal limits of nursing. Although California had enlarged the scope of nursing practice in a revised Nursing Practice Act in 1974, it did not refer to nurses practicing independently. The American Nurses' Association had enlarged the nurse's role in "The Scope of Nursing Practice" and in "Standards: Psychiatric-Mental Health Nursing." My educational preparation qualified me as a clinical nurse specialist in psychiatric-mental health nursing. Most nurses with my background worked in a hospital, clinic, or educational system.

I was rescued from resolving the latter dilemma by a temporary change in the criteria for Marriage, Family, Child Counselor (MFCC) licensing to include nurses with a master's degree in psychiatric nursing. I applied and qualified to sit for the state licensing examination. I received my license in 1976. Unfortunately, I was still faced with the financial dilemma because MFCCs also were unsuccessful in receiving insurance reimbursement. By this time I had come in contact with two nurses who had successfully established private practices in psychiatric-mental health nursing with self-paying clients. I felt more optimistic, but still had to go about my own transition.

I wanted to combine my experience with orthopedics, my interest in problems of pain and loss with my psychiatric background. I was placed in a unique position when I underwent orthopedic surgery. I was able to demonstrate and discuss pain relief techniques with my physician. I provided him with a potential solution to a problem he had with patients who were unresponsive to customary medical treatment. We negotiated a trial period for me to see patients with chronic pain part time. I continued my teaching job. The major hurdle to overcome was financial feasibility. The patients I would see were injured workers. Workers' (formerly known as "Workmen's") compensation carriers must authorize treatment before they will pay the provider of service. Thus, we had to test the insurance companies to see if they would authorize me to see patients I was referred. This process required much explanation and clarification, but I received sufficient authorization to shift to a full-time commitment after a three-month trial period.

Overcoming the Obstacles

The next few years were a mixture of pain, insecurity, and tremendous growth. I was unprepared for independent practice and functioning within the workers' compensation system, and consequently, I encountered some problems. They fall into three categories: independent practice, consultant role with physicians, and adjustment to the worker's compensation system.

Problems of Independent Practice

In practicing independently, my major problem areas were maintaining financial records, paying taxes, time management, and isolation. I had become used to the convenience of my employer withholding taxes and keeping my financial records. In my new role, I was paid a fee for service. My patient fees went into a corporation and I billed the corporation a fee based on my records of service. The remainder of the patient fee was retained by the corporation to cover billing, answering service, transcribing, rent, secretarial costs, and so on. I was so naive about this whole process that I was late paying my first tax estimate because I didn't know taxes must be paid quarterly for wages subject to withholding tax. I also had to apply for a tax identification number and business license. I was shocked to find out I had to pay Social Security at the end of each year. Needless to say, I found that I benefited from the assistance of an accountant.

When I was employed by a hospital or university, I was paid a salary for either performing a job description or teaching specified courses. My use of time was dictated by the circumstances of my employment. As long as I completed the course or put in my time, I received my pay. I was paid when sick or on vacation. I soon learned what a luxury that arrangement is. On my own I quickly realized "time is money." Time not involved with a patient was time without income. I had to become much more disciplined about lengths of phone conversations, discussions with physicians, insurance companies, and so on regarding patients. My priorities were my patients' appointments, patient-related activities (data collection and communication), record keeping, and public relations to help generate referrals. Personal contact with physicians and insurance-carrier representatives was vital. In addition, I work with staff nurses when my patients are hospitalized. Vacations meant loss of income so I chose to take long weekends, holidays, and a week off quarterly. I still must become much more disciplined in time management, especially in keeping up with my business records.

The longest lasting problem I encountered was isolation. I worked with physical therapists, physicians, and vocational rehabilitation counselors. A few nurses I knew were in private practice, but primarily dealt with a very different type of patient. My patients always had an active physical disability involving pain accompanied by emotional and social problems. For two and a half years I had only one colleague with knowledge and interests similar to mine; she also was a nurse. I found it very difficult not having anyone to share assessment and intervention techniques with. Physicians provided role models for functioning in the workers' compensation system. I received valued personal support from several nurse friends and a kinesiologist with whom I worked, but I missed having a connection with others who had skill and experience in my area of specialization. Fortunately, I found what I was looking for while receiving training in biofeedback. All my instructors worked with psychophysiological conditions. What a joy that was to feel connected again! Sadly, not one of these individuals was a nurse.

Problems of the Consultant Role

By working as a consultant initially in pain management, I had to communicate closely with the referring physician because the patient was still under medical treatment. I saw the patient either one time for evaluation and recommendations or first for an initial evaluation and then for pain management. I was referred patients primarily by two orthopedic surgeons and two neurosurgeons. At first I was met with varying degrees of acceptance, even blatant skepticism. It was an interesting process to see the most skeptical physician turn out to be a great ally and best at identifying and referring patients I could help. Some physicians referred their most frustrating and chronically disabled patients.

In this new role, I soon identified a number of ineffective responses with which I had been socialized.

I had become conditioned to report my observations along with many justifications for their accuracy or validity. I had tremendous difficulty reaching conclusions and giving recommendations. I was too wordy. I thought back to all the emphasis nursing schools and hospitals placed on assessment and information gathering, but how little they placed on conclusions and recommendations. Suddenly, I was being faced with accountability and going beyond data gathering. The physicians didn't want all the descriptions and justifications, they just wanted to know what I thought should be done. This habit was hard to break; I was regularly asked to be brief and to the point. I actually had to justify my conclusions far more to nurses.

One cause for my wordiness was a reticence to arrive at conclusions on patients after only one interview. I was fearful of arriving at incorrect conclusions. Again, in nursing we do not gain experience in taking a stand where nursing interventions are concerned or we'd see explicit nursing care plans or nursing orders being followed by nursing staff. I went through the process of taking the risk and being desensitized to the fear of making a mistake.

Another concern that increased my cautiousness was an attempt to avoid criticism, putdowns, or disagreement, particularly with the physicians. I eventually learned that much of my sensitivity was coming from my belief that I was being picked on because I am a nurse and/or female and thus not a peer. To my amazement, when I observed the interactions objectively, I found that my treatment was no different from the way one physician questioned or disagreed with another. It was enormously valuable for me to work closely with four physicians to see the way they dealt with one another. I suggest strongly to nurses that, when communicating your opinion to a physician, you not take the response you receive personally. Deal with it in a nondefensive manner.

Overall, the experience of having to communicate closely with physicians in a consultant role has been extremely beneficial to my self-confidence. I am so used to saying what I think and making recommendations that I only notice the change when dealing with physicians with whom I've had little contact. Sometimes I receive a confused or hesitant response. Generally, however, I did not encounter problems. Where my management of the patient was involved, I encountered no interference. I was entirely able to carry out what I wanted to do. The only areas of conflict occurred where the physician disagreed with my recommendations for prescribing or carrying out procedures or treatment that fell clearly into the domain of medical practice. Although my recommendations were frequently followed, disagreements were inevitable. After all, I also disagreed with recommendations made by the treating physician for treatment falling into my area of specialization. The important issue here was that we based our decisions on our judgment of what was indicated, not on irrational responses to a doctor-nurse game.

Problems in Adjusting to the Workers' Compensation System

My adjustment to working with the workers' compensation system was an ongoing process. In general, all aspects of my work with patients were more difficult because of it. The major benefit was that I could receive full payment for my services. The worker's compensation carriers did not discriminate against me for being a nurse as did the private carriers. In each state there are laws pertaining to the type and amount of assistance an injured worker receives. In California, laws require that the worker receive medical treatment, tax-free wage replacement, permanent disability if indicated, and vocational rehabilitation if the worker is medically eligible and it is vocationally feasible. When treatment is completed, the physical condition of the patient is rated by the physician as to limitations and percentage of permanent disability. These ratings form the basis of settlements and limitations in future work. Many variables come into play in assessing an injured worker's condition. Many aspects of symptomatology are subjective (e.g., pain, sensory changes, limitation of motion and strength); other findings are considered objective (e.g., reflex loss, EMG and x-ray results). There is tremendous room for error with subjective symptoms and much medical disagreement on the significance of the objective findings. These inconsistencies are importent in workers' compensation, where decisions must be made on the type and length of treatment, duration of temporary disability, ability of the patient to return to usual employment, and monetary settlements.

The system itself is aimed at helping the injured worker recover and return to work. Unlike most medical treatment, the goal of treatment and measure of success is return to work. The injured worker's case is supervised by a claims examiner. The background and experience of claims representatives vary greatly. Many have limited knowledge regarding appropriate medical treatment. A number of insurance carriers provide education and case reviews to reduce misinformation. Some claims examiners are very cynical; others, very concerned. Most have large case loads. Often their job of supervising cases and deciding whether or not to authorize treatment is hampered by the unavailability of the injured worker's (also known as claimant) insurance file. I feel that claims examiners have a very difficult job.

Often the tone and type of service provided for the claimant are set by the insurance carrier. Some are well organized and have devised ways to identify cases that may require particular attention and aggressive treatment to prevent chronicity. Others are very disorganized, to the point of filing charts by keeping them piled on rows on tables. Increasingly, carriers are utilizing nurses to help monitor and coordinate treatment, make personal contact with patients, assist rehabilitation, and clarify medical information for nonmedical staff. In my experience, treatment runs more smoothly and patients are usually less dissatisfied when rehabilitation nurses are involved. Finally, some insurance carriers refuse to authorize any care identified as outside standard medical treatment. They refuse any referrals for pain management techniques, for example. One company sent me a letter stating they would not authorize any referrals to me and cautioned me that I would not be paid if I worked with any of their claimants.

That example provides an appropriate transition to the reason some patients seek legal advice. Attorneys are prevalent in the workers' compensation system. Easily three-fourths of my patients were represented by attorneys. Some attorneys were very helpful to their clients, helping them obtain adequate care, temporary disability payments, and so forth. Others sent clients for multiple consultations to build a case for settlement. In some cases, the patient received practically no treatment; in other cases the patient's treatment was palliative and not aimed at recovery. I have worked with a number of patients who were in need of treatment and had become sidetracked by the potential of money. One of the most blatant examples associating injury with settlement is the top line of an ad that regularly appears in a local newspaper. In bold type the ad states, "PAIN—INJURY— MONEY." This type of advertising is frowned upon by many attorneys. There were situations where the stress of the system was reduced and treatment facilitated by caring attorneys, especially when the claimant-insurance carrier relationship had deteriorated. I have seen situations where the attorney-referred physicians or other medical professionals and the insurance carrier-referred physicians totally disagreed on medical management, disability status, and ability to return to work. The patients were caught in the middle, confused and becoming distrustful. Many patients had preconceived notions that the insurance company treatment referrals hold allegiances to the insurance carrier, not to the patient.

Very often, the injured workers I saw had been employed in heavy labor or engaged in some type of physical activity on the job. Statistically, the most common injury causing lost work time is to the back. The worker is frequently male, between the ages of thirty-nine and forty-five. Many of the individuals I saw had relied on physical strength as a way to earn a good salary. Once injured, my patients' income on temporary disability was usually no greater than maximum wage replacement, $152/week unless they were covered by another policy allowing them some type of salary continuation. In addition, a number of the claimants were unable to return to heavy work because of the injury. Unfortunately, most job alternatives not physically demanding commonly pay close to mininum wage. Many of the patients had gone into debt while on disability and were faced with a career change resulting in lower pay at middle age.

Some patients decide for varying reasons that it's best to aim for a settlement or job retraining because of dissatisfaction, anger, retirement, or other factors. Motivation to improve symptoms in some injured workers is very low because goals of settlement or retraining can't be met if symptoms improve. Others somehow get caught in the complex system and develop chronic symptoms.

All these variables and more operated with each patient I was referred. When I started seeing patients, most of them had been disabled two to six years. They usually had multiple problems that were extremely complex to deal with. Often the patients had no particular desire to come for the first visit. Many were suspicious that a referral to me meant that their physical symptoms were in question. A number of patients were angry and bitter about their circumstances. On some occasions, a patient was informed by the insurance carrier that disability payments would be withheld until they came in for a consultation. I rarely saw a patient who was not initially suspicious, angry, or bitter. A nondefensive approach on my part was a necessity.

The most difficult aspect for me in dealing with the patients was coming to grips with the reality that some people will be deceitful and willing to embellish symptoms or maintain disability. I did find true malingerers to be rare, however. Most patients did in fact have physical problems. I found that I had to develop a structure to my evaluation process in order to avoid developing the cynicism so prevalent in workers' compensation. I gradually identified criteria to use in helping me decide if I could work with a particular patient. There are many factors involved in response to treatment and a list of patient's losses versus gains from the injury and system is beneficial. Communication with claims examiners and rehabilitation nurses was essential in the smooth running of the case. Coordinating treatment and educating the insurance representative and patient regarding findings and goals decreased confusion and distrust. The ideal situation was to have all parties involved working together in a coordinated fashion. In this situation, the focus isn't only the nurse/patient relationship. It is enormously beneficial to reduce the adversary nature of the workers' compensation system.

The most frustrating adjustment to workers' compensation other than patient-related issues was dictating reports. Once a patient was seen for consultation, a report detailing the evaluation, conclusion, and recommendations had to be sent to the insurance carrier; a copy was also sent to the treating physician. If I had problems verbally arriving at conclusions that were brief and to the point, imagine what happened when I had to produce this information in a typed report.

These reports could be sent to anyone involved in the patient's case and could even be subpoenaed. Besides my reluctance to put my opinions in writing, I had no experience dictating. I had the additional problem of having to develop the format for my report. My evaluation did not fit the standard nursing, medical, or psychological formats for assessment. My first report was twelve typewritten pages, and I wrote it out in longhand before I dictated it. Shortly thereafter I dictated rough drafts from notes because writing out reports was too time-consuming. I then proofread the typed rough draft and dictated the final copy from it. While I was struggling with dictating, I revised my evaluation format many times. For approximately one year, I was reluctant to dictate a report following an initial consultation. I felt I needed to know more about how the patient would respond before taking a position in a report. I think I was concerned about the insurance carrier discontinuing authorization if the claimant's progress didn't match my initial estimates. I felt pressure to prove myself. I finally learned the technique of making decisions based on available information. I cannot stress enough the importance of learning this skill. It helps bridge the gap between gathering data and drawing conclusions. Treatment of a patient does not have to be disorganized and tentative just because I don't know everything there is to know about that person. Thus, I began to produce reports soon after initial evaluation and modified my conclusions and recommendations as new information became available.

In my struggle with dictating reports, I have learned ways to facilitate progress. Try out different machines if at all possible; identify the characteristics that make one easier and more convenient to use. I found that machines that allow rapid review of dictation and ease in correcting errors or rewording sentences very helpful. Having a format to follow when dictating is a must. Organize the patient interview in the same sequence as the format for dictation. Incorporate all the information available into the format. By maintaining a set sequence, comfortable wording and skeletons of paragraphs that can be used repeatedly begin to develop. With repetition they flow easily from memory; only the specific details for each patient need to be added from notations. When actually dictating, it is beneficial to create a ritual or routine. This might include selecting a specific location; having music or something to drink; checking to be sure notes are complete and easily located and all information is at hand; and controlling interruption. On several occasions, I have been in the middle of a report and couldn't locate a test report or some other needed information. That wastes time and interrupts the flow of words. Finally, be prepared for the discomfort of progressing from writing reports longhand to dictating rough drafts to dictating final copies from notes; most people have to pressure themselves to make the transition. Also, many people dislike the act of dictating reports. I found that dictating helped me organize my thoughts and become more concise in my wording. My initial reports are now five typewritten pages long.

The most recent dilemma I have experienced was having my reports subpoenaed. My greatest revelation was to find that I was surprised anyone other than the referring physician would find my opinion of value. I was in complete disbelief when I was subpoenaed to testify at a trial. The old nursing identity problems had emerged. What could I possibly say that would be given the weight of a physician's testimony? I was also concerned that I not misrepresent my legal boundaries as a nurse. Although I was apprehensive, I resolved much of my fear by talking with people who have testified and clarifying my role with the client's attorney. As it turned out, the parties settled out of court. I had accomplished another shift toward improving my identity as a nurse.

Reflection

Although I have experienced growing pains and frustration over my lack of preparation in dealing with independent practice, I must emphasize how worthwhile the experience has been. I had to undergo very stressful times, but I do not think I could have gained so much in personal and professional growth without it. The workers' compensation system provided a feedback loop for evaluating many of my skills, particularly in the areas of assessing, arriving at conclusions and recommendations for treatment, dictating, and finally maintaining a critical view of my management of patients. Feedback was continuous, thus allowing regular corrective moves on my part. Since payment was not an issue, I also was able to work with a wide variety of patients in much larger numbers than would be possible in other areas of private practice. My patients crossed all socioeconomic and racial groups. I learned so much from them. My psychiatric-mental health skills have vastly improved. This experience has given me confidence in myself that I did not possess in 1977 when I began consulting. I would not want to return to employee status. I enjoy the control and freedom I have developed even though hard work is involved. Starting January 1981, I qualified for private insurance reimbursement under my MFCC license. I am freer to see patients not under workers' compensation and plan to increase the number of private patients I see. This option allows me to work more often with patients having psychophysiological conditions such as essential hypertension. Since the type of patient I most often see requires periodic medical management, I am continuing my close association with physicians. My referral sources, however, have expanded to family practice physicians, internists, and gynecologists. I am looking forward to continued growth and excitement in my practice of nursing, certainly an enormous departure from my years of frustration.

References

American Nurses' Association. *The Scope of Nursing Practice.* Kansas City, Missouri: 1976.

American Nurses' Association. *Standards: Psychiatric Mental Health Nursing Practice.* Kansas City, Missouri: 1973.

Part B

Foundations for Establishing Your Own Business

8

A Legal Overview

Julie Bornstein

One cannot begin a business without some concern for the legal ramifications. This chapter attempts to examine the legal effects of various forms of doing business as well as to provide "tips" to the new business that may help it avoid certain pitfalls affecting its eventual success.

Prior to beginning a business, one must make decisions as to the legal form that business will take. Still other decisions must be made concerning the way in which the business is to be conducted, which can greatly enhance or negate the efforts of the business owner in ensuring success. There are three general forms of doing business, which are common to most states, and which should be considered in the formation of any new business. These are corporations, partnerships, and proprietorships. Each form will be discussed in some detail.

The author is a California lawyer and any comments made in this chapter are based on the education and experience of an attorney practicing California law. Most of the comments are general in nature and are given as a guide to the person preparing to open a business. Certainly any general advice given should be used in conjunction with advice obtained in consultation with a lawyer in the state in which the business is to be formed, and a tax adviser well versed in both state and federal taxation. The advice given in this chapter is therefore general in nature, and should not be relied upon exclusively in the formation of a business.

The Corporation

Almost anyone may form a corporation. The states differ in how many persons are required to do so, but there are no other major limitations. It is therefore quite easy for almost any businessperson to become president and chairman of the board of a corporation! The questions to be asked in forming a corporation are more important, however, than the title that goes on the business card. One should thoroughly understand the ramifications of incorporating before making that decision, and a comparison should be made by anyone starting a new business as to the major advantages and disadvantages of the business forms available prior to incorporating.

A corporation is a separate legal entity. When a corporation is formed, it has the same legal consequence as the birth of a new person. The corporation has an existence, separate from the person or persons forming it. Since a corporation itself is not a person, it must act through others. A corporation therefore makes its legal commitments through the actions of its officers and directors. When a person is acting as an officer and/or director of a corporation, that capacity should be designated so that all legal documents are clear in their intent. Ownership in a corporation is in the shareholders. The rights and responsibilities of the shareholders are different from those of the officers and directors, although many times the shareholders and the officers and directors are the same people, especially in a small corporation. One must be aware of the different hats one must wear in forming a corporation, so that all the legal advantages of a corporation are maintained. Each state differs in how important it is to follow the legal formalities required by incorporation. It is very important to check into the laws in your state to determine what formalities are required. One of the disadvantages of a corporation is the necessity of additional paperwork as well as certain other formal requirements to maintain a separate identity of a corporation. Certain states also require a minimum annual tax payment, California for instance requiring $200 a year. One of the advantages, however, of doing business in corporate form is that maintaining a separate legal entity protects personal assets of the shareholders from creditors if the business is unsuccessful. It is therefore evident that in order to maintain that advantage one must conform with the appropriate state laws.

To form a corporation, the person or persons who wish to begin a new business must file the necessary Articles of Incorporation. Many times Articles of Incorporation are filed under the names of persons who are not directly involved in the business, either to expedite the filing of those Articles or to prevent the public record from reflecting the true ownership of the company. The content of the Articles of Incorporation is usually dictated by state law, and very little variation is required or desired. This document is the paper that "gives birth" to the new legal entity. Once the Articles of Incorporation are filed, the corporation is in existence, but certain other documents must be drafted and accepted before it is fully functioning. The most important of these documents is the bylaws, which set forth a general procedure under which the corporation is governed. This procedure is common to almost every business corporation and involves how many persons are required for a quorum, the term of office of the officers and directors, the number of officers and directors, and the establishment of rights of minority shareholders. The bylaws should be presented to the directors as soon after incorporation as practical and adopted upon presentation.

In order for the bylaws to be presented and adopted, of course, the directors and officers must be elected. Remember, a corporation can only act through its officers and directors, and therefore no action can be taken until those persons have been elected and assume the duties of office. It is therefore also necessary to have a meeting of directors and/or shareholders as soon after incorporation as practical. At that first meeting a number of important items of business must take place. The officers and directors must be nominated and elected and must accept their positions. The corporation must adopt certain resolutions to provide for the banking for the corporation's business. The corporation must adopt a share certificate, authorize he officers to cooperate in the issuance of the share certificates, and adopt the corporate seal. The corporation must establish its principal place of business, and its accounting year for tax purposes. The corporation must also authorize the officers and directors to take any other action so that business may begin. In particular, then, the corporation must be authorized through the actions of its officers and directors to conform with any local and state licensing laws, so that the profession of the corporation may be practiced in conformance with the law. All these actions must be duly authorized by the corporation or they may be later set aside if challenged by outsiders.

Therefore, in order to have a corporation formed and functioning in business, one must file Articles of Incorporation, create and adopt bylaws, and hold a meeting for which minutes are taken that establish the very basic authority of the officers and directors and commence the business. Thereafter, if you are doing business in a corporate form, you will need to memorialize all major actions to some written corporate resolution or through minutes of meetings of the corporation. Such actions include paying yourself a salary, adopting pension, profit-sharing, or medical reimbursement plans, entering into a lease, changing the principal place of business of the corporation, and changing the location of your banking.

If this seems like a lot of extra paperwork, you might ask yourself why people wish to do business in a corporate form. The answer is complicated and depends on the personal circumstances of the business owner.

Advantages and Disadvantages

The most common reason to do business in the corporate form is the desire to limit liabilities. For example, if a person has been successful in building up a certain number of assets, whether they be a home, money in the bank, or other property, he or she may not wish to risk those assets in a new business venture. By doing business in the corporate form—assuming one follows all the corporate formalities required by state law—the business owner can limit his or her liabilities to the property owned by the corporation. In other words, if you originally put $10,000 into your corporation for the purchase of stock, and your business does not do well and you ultimately owe $15,000, the creditors of the corporation look only to the corporation for satisfaction of their debts; they may have to take a pro rata reduction of their debts upon the corporation's bankruptcy, dissolution, or insolvency. Thus, if you have other assets you wish to protect, a major reason for choosing the corporate form is to insulate your own assets from liability for corporate debts. When undertaking a new business, this is one advantage of a corporation that should be considered.

Another reason to choose the corporate form is the fact that it lives forever, and its interests are easily transferable. If you wish to start a business now and you think that if the business is successful you may wish to bring in other investors, or that you might wish to sell the business and take your profits in that manner, a corporation may be a desirable mode to select. Since a corporation ownership is reflected by shares, and shares may be sold (so long as you comply with the state laws regarding the transfer of stock), it is easy to bring in additional investors, or to sell all your stock in a corporation by simply selling the shares. The corporation continues under the same name, in the same location, and with the same employees if desired. Thus a corporate ownership also allows for easy transferability of ownership interest.

Depending on your own particular tax situation, a corporation may be a desirable form of doing business, because the tax laws allow an owner to be treated as an employee and receive certain benefits. In other words, you may own all the stock in a corporation, but since you are also an employee you receive the benefits of certain pension plans and medical reimbursement plans. The other side of this coin, however, is that to pay yourself a salary you must also withhold taxes from your own salary as if you were any other employee. The decision to incorporate is largely a tax decision, and should be made in conjunction with your tax adviser as regards your own particular situation. *A major mistake* made by many small business owners is that they incorporate because they have heard from friends that it is the thing to do, without consulting their tax adviser as to whether it is beneficial to their own tax picture. A corporation can have many tax advantages for the owner, but it can also have disadvantages inasmuch as any income received by the corporation is taxed first when received by the corporation, and then it is taxed again when received by the individual either as salary or as dividends on stock. This is referred to as double taxation, and is one disadvantage of a corporation. Table 8-1 compares the advantages and disadvantages of different forms of doing business.

The corporate form is, therefore, not for everyone. It does require additional paperwork to conform with state law concerning corporate formalities. Although corporate form may give certain tax advantages to some shareholders, it provides double taxation to others. The corporate form of doing business does not eliminate any of the other requirements of doing business, which are necessary to conform with state and local laws and applicable to all businesses. Thus, the business owner must be aware of the advantages and disadvantages before choosing the corporate form, because once one gives birth to this new entity, certain other procedures must be followed to provide it a decent burial if one chooses to cease doing business in a corporate form.

The Partnership

There are two types of partnerships in most states: general partnerships and limited partnerships. In a general partnership, all the partners to the partnership have general liability for all the debts and actions of the partnership, and are able to bind the partnership as well as have a hand in the daily management and control of partnership business. A limited partnership must meet certain other formalities. Limited partners have limited liability, whereas the general partner or partners of the limited partnership have general liability for the debts of the business, as well as the complete control of the management of the business. In exchange for their limited liability, limited partners have *no say* in the daily operation of the business. Very often limited partners are called *silent partners.*

A partnership may be a new business entity, but it is not necessarily a new legal entity. The distinction is important in understanding what happens to the assets of the individual partners when the debts of the partnership business exceed the partnership assets. If two persons who decide to open a business have no written agreement between them, have equal control of the management of the business, and appear to be the owners of the business, even without that written agreement they have formed a general partnership. Certainly it is advisable from many points of view to have a written agreement, so that the partners understand their obligations and rights, and so that the outside world, if it is required to examine the partnership, is aware of what the agreement between the parties actually is. Most states do not require a written agreement to form a general partnership, and persons must be careful that they do not form one by accident. A general partnership does not necessarily imply that all partners have an equal interest. In other words, just because there are two partners it does not mean that each partner owns 50 percent of the business. The percentage interest of the partners in the business may be varied according to the agreements of the parties. In addition, just because one person puts in 25 percent of the capital and the other 75 percent does not mean that the business is owned one-fourth and three-fourths, respectively.

For these reasons, it is advisable to have a written agreement. In the written partnership agreement, the partners may specify how much they are each contributing in capital, and what percentage interest each holds in the ownership of the business as a result. The written agreement should also specify how the profits and losses are divided and whether the partnership survives the death or disability of any of the partners. Technically speaking, a partnership may have any number of partners but caution should be taken if the number exceeds ten because the partnership may fall under the jurisdiction of certain state and national securities regulations, and to comply requires additional expense and time.

A partnership, once it is formed and a written agreement is signed, does not thereafter require all the formalities of a corporation. One need not register with the local secretary of state, nor file yearly statements of officers and directors. The partnership may act by its partners, and does not require written resolutions or elections of officers and directors to confirm and ratify actions of the business. State and certainly federal tax laws do not require double taxation of partnership business, and partnership losses may be used to offset income from other sources. However, the other side of the coin is that certain tax benefits of corporations are not available to partnerships.

Generally speaking, it is much easier to conduct business in the partnership form than in the corporation form because less attention must be given to the legal formalities and more attention can be devoted to the actual conduct of business. If the partners are satisfied with the tax effects of a partnership and are willing to place all their personal assets on the line for the conduct of the business, the partnership form should be considered.

The most important thing to the creation of a partnership is, of course, the selection of the partner. I am not the first to state that a partnership is like a marriage, and the same care that goes into the selection of a marital partner should be given to the selection of a business partner. A major mistake made by many people is that they select their best friend as their business partner. This is not always the most appropriate selection. A business partner must have the same attitude toward work, the practice of the profession, the hiring and firing of personnel, and most generally the handling of money, so that the partnership can function smoothly. Although it might be fun to work with one's best friend on a daily basis, it is not the best business decision. This is especially true when that best friend likes to take time off for personal matters when the business requires the full-time attention of both parties, or when one partner wants to take certain risks and reinvest the profits of the business to expand it, and the other partner is more conservative and wants to build up the partnership bank account instead. Needless to say, no business is going to do well if the partners are fighting between themselves over decisions about the general direction of the business. Because partners have the same management and control over the business, it is therefore vitally important that the proper selection of a partner be made.

Limited Partnership

Much is misunderstood about the limited partnership, where one can take in a silent partner. Limited partnerships are established by law in most states, and many states have adopted the Uniform Limited Partnership Act. A limited partnership must have a written agreement, so that the outside world is aware of the limited liability of the limited partners. A limited partner puts in a specified amount of capital and risks nothing more than that. In other words, liability is limited. If a business is formed where the limited partners each contribute $10,000 and that business fails, owing $60,000, the limited partners are not at risk for anything more than their original $10,000 investment. In exchange for that limited liability, they simply must sit back and act as investors and have no control over the day-to-day affairs of the partnership. The laws in each state vary, but most states allow the limited partners only to have the right to remove and replace the general partner under certain conditions.

Every limited partnership has two classes of partners, as we have seen: the limited partners, as described in the previous paragraph, and the general partner. Again, there is no maximum number of partners set by law, but one must be careful that if there are too many investors the partnership may become subject to certain securities regulations thus increasing the cost and legal formality of doing business. The general partner is charged with the conduct and management of the partnership business. The general partner also has general liability and is therefore responsible for all the debts of the partnership over and above the capital of the partnership. Thus, if a partnership dissolves, leaving $60,000 in debts, with the limited partners having contributed a total of $30,000, the general partner and the general partner's personal assets are liable for the remaining $30,000. A limited partnership form may be desirable if one wishes to start a business but is short of capital and has willing and trusting investors ready to invest. Because the partners participating are investors, they are not limited by any state usury laws as to the amount of return they might get if they had lent the money rather than invested it. On the other hand, if the business does not do well there is no obligation on the part of the general partners to repay the money, since all partners are investors in the business. Thus the limited partners are taking the risk with the general partner that the business will do well, although their risk is limited to the amount of capital they are investing.

To form a limited partnership one must have a written limited partnership agreement, specifying all the rights and obligations of each of the partners, the capital contribution of all the partners, the duties of the general partner, a statement that the limited partners do have limited liability, and the percentage distribution of profits and losses. Many times it is also advisable to file a Certificate of Limited Partnership with the local county recorder. Filing is required if the business ever owns or leases real property where the lease is recorded. Other than these written documents, the limited partnership is no more complicated in operation than a general partnership, so long as the limited partners understand that they can have no participation in the management and control of the partnership business. Thus partnerships, both general and limited, provide for multiparty ownership of a business without the formalities, complications, tax consequences, and in some cases limited liability of the corporation.

The Proprietorship

In the sole proprietorship, a single person owns a business and operates that business as the sole owner. There is no separate level of taxation or legal entity other than the individual. All income made by the individual in the business is charged to that individual directly, and all deductions taken by the business are again offset by that individual against income from all sources. The assets of the individual stand behind all the debts of the business and there is no insulation from liability whatsoever. A proprietorship is easy to form and operate, since it requires no written agreement, and no selection of other persons with whom to do the business. All decisions are therefore made by the sole owner without consultation with anyone else being required. Most small businesses owned by a single owner start off as a sole proprietorship and, upon reaching a certain level of success, and based upon the advice of the accountant and lawyer of the business, later on become corporations.

The disadvantages of a proprietorship might be the same as those of a general partnership. There is no insulation from liability for the debts of the business against the personal assets of the business owner, and certain tax benefits available to corporations are not available to the proprietor. This form of doing business has the fewest legal formalities and is therefore the simplest way to conduct business, so that the owner's attention is more directly related to the actual conduct of business.

General Business Requirements

Common to all businesses are the following requirements:

1. A separate taxpayer identification number should be applied for by the business and obtained so that employment taxes, income taxes, and other tax information derived only from the business may be kept separate from the personal affairs of the business owners.

2. A fictitious name statement must be prepared, filed, and recorded. A fictitious name statement is a statement by a business owner that a business is being conducted under a name other than that of the business owner. Since most businesses do not conduct business under the actual personal name of the owner, this is a requirement applicable to most businesses. It does not matter whether the business is being conducted by a corporation, a partnership, or an individual, and it is advisable under most circumstances. A fictitious name statement is usually a preprinted form that must be filled out and filed according to the directions on the statement. These forms are available from many different sources according to your locality, and your attorney or the county clerk will be able to tell you where to get them. In most states it must be renewed every five years or so. The purpose of a fictitious name statement is to let the rest of the world know who the actual owner of a business is. Although this may initially offend the sensibilities of one desiring to do business under a fictitious name, consider its logic. Some individuals may attempt to hide from their creditors by doing business under a fictitious name, and it is only fair to allow those creditors to know how the business is conducted (in what form) and who is responsible for the payment of debts. There is usually a nominal filing fee charged for the filing and recording of a fictitious name statement.

3. All businesses must pay employment taxes when they employ people to whom a salary is paid. These employment taxes apply whether the business is a proprietorship, a partnership, or a corporation. In a corporation, of course, all persons working in a business are employees, even the owner of the business. When the employer tax number is obtained, owners of a business will receive state and local tax information, which should give adequate directions on when to make deposits and file returns. Also, booklets listing withholding schedules should be mailed, and if they are not received shortly after business is begun and employees hired, a telephone call to the local taxing authority should provide the needed information.

It is *vital* to comply with all tax laws concerning employee taxes. Too many young businesses get into trouble because employee taxes are not paid at the right times. Late taxes incur penalties and interest, and most young businesses can ill afford to pay money in that manner. Also, criminal penalties exist on the books in most states for the nonpayment of employee taxes in a timely manner, and certainly if they are intentionally withheld and not paid to the state. Unnecessary legal expenses can therefore be avoided by knowing the employee tax laws and complying with them in a timely manner.

4. A separate bank account should be maintained for the business, regardless of the form of doing business. Certainly if the objective of the business owner is to insulate liability, one can see that the banking of the business should be kept separate from the personal affairs of the business owner. From an accounting standpoint, it is much easier to separate business expenses from personal expenses. This means not paying one's rent check out of the business bank account, and not paying business expenses with a personal check. This might seem like more bookkeeping at the outset, but at the end of your first tax year you will be thankful that you have conducted your business in this way when you see the lower accounting bill you receive than a friend who has done it differently. Thus regardless of the form of doing business, separate bank accounts should be maintained for the business, and all personal affairs should be handled by personal banking accounts.

A corollary to the maintenance of separate bank accounts for personal and business matters is the suggestion that separate credit cards be utilized by the business. A common bone of contention with the Internal Revenue Service is whether certain entertainment expenses were incurred for business or personal use. If the business has a separate credit card on which all business expenses are charged, and receipts are kept, it is much easier to convince the IRS auditor that those expenses are all business related—even if the receipt is lost at the time of the audit. On the other hand, if the business owner uses one credit card for both business and personal matters, it requires extensive bookkeeping to separate the different charges, either at the end of each month or at the end of a year. Thus the initial work of applying for two separate cards and paying two bills on a monthly basis is justified by the long-range benefits. This also means that to review business entertainment expenses for the year, one would simply have to look at the totals for that account, without making any deductions for personal expenses. Thus the maintenance bank and credit records for business and personal affairs is definitely suggested. It is even more important if there is more than one owner in the business, so that neither owner feels that the other is taking more personal expenses out of business funds. Many a lawsuit has been fought between former partners concerning the expenditure of business funds for personal obligations.

Table 8-1 compares the advantages and disadvantages of the different forms of business organizations discussed in this chapter. A careful analysis of these factors in consultation with legal and tax advisers should go a long way toward suggesting the appropriate legal entity for your business.

Table 8.1 Characteristics of the Different Forms of Business

	Corpo-ration	Partnership General	Limited	Proprietorship
Number of owners	One or more	Two or more	Two or more	One
Legal formalities	Most	Some	More	Fewest
Separate tax-payer number	Yes	Yes	Yes	Yes
Insulation from			Yes for limited	No
Double tax-ation of	Yes	No	partner	
income	Yes	No	No	No
How ownership is held	Shares	Partnership interest	General or limited partnership interest	Direct ownership of assets
Management of business by	Officers	Partners	General partner	Owner

Other Business Suggestions

Although legal expenses are a recognized business expense, most beginning businesses can ill afford to spend a lot of money for legal fees. Certain preventive steps can be taken by the new business owner to keep the legal fees required to a minumum. This means knowing rights and obligations as a business owner so as to avoid legal difficulties affecting a new business.

One major element has already been discussed. The business owner should be familiar with the obligations regarding taxes and workers' compensation insurance so that legal advice is not required to conform with the laws. It is better to consult an attorney at the beginning of the business so that one may fully understand one's legal obligations, rather than to try to avoid a relatively small expense at the beginning in the hopes that it will all work out in the end. If a new business owner does not understand all the tax and legal obligations required by municipalities in the state in which the business is located, the appropriate professional should be consulted to obtain the necessary information. Most governmental authorities have the ability to impose penalties and interest, and may bring either civil or criminal legal action against the employer for failure to conform with the appropriate laws. No one likes to start out their business career as a defendant in a criminal action for nonpayment of employer taxes! The legal fees in connection with such a defense are certainly greater than any legal fees that might be incurred at the outset by way of consultation to understand the taxing obligations.

Leases and rental agreements should also be reviewed by an attorney prior to signature. In most areas attorneys charge relatively low fees for reviewing documents and advising on the contents. If, on the other hand, the initial fees are "saved" and the lease entered into later turns out to be unfavorable to the tenant, many more dollars may be spent in the long run. A word of caution should also be given to those operating a business under a fictitious name, a partnership, or a corporation. One must make sure that the legal entity signing the lease or rental agreement is the owner of the business and the actual occupant of the space. In other words, if you are doing business in a corporate form, the corporation should sign the lease; if you are doing business in the partnership form, the name of the partnership should sign the lease. Do not be surprised, however, if the landlord also requires each partner to sign the lease or a personal guarantee by the corporation shareholders. Unless the corporation itself has sufficient assets and credit to justify being the sole signatory to the lease, the individuals behind the corporation may also be asked to assume that liability. That is not an uncommon practice for a beginning business, and will only take away the corporate insulation of liability for the document actually signed by the individuals.

It is also suggested that a written document of some kind be signed with all customers or users of your services. The reasons for this are many. First, it is always a good idea to have the relationship between you and your customers clearly stated. This means that you will clearly state what product or services are to be provided and they will clearly understand the limitations of your service. It should also be clearly stated how payments are to be made and the price to be paid. That way each party understands their obligations under the business relationship for the provision of services. Second, if there should be a disagreement between the parties, this can be easily solved by either lawyers examining the documents or a court if a lawsuit results. The documents should then clearly state what is being provided, what is being charged, and how the charge is to be paid. Third, in most jursidictions a party who prevails in a lawsuit cannot collect the amount of its attorney's fees in bringing that lawsuit unless the right is provided by contract or statute. This can become vitally important to your business. If you agree to provide a service to a customer for a charge of $500 and the customer fails to pay, you do not want to have to incur $450 in attorneys' fees to collect that debt, for the net results will of course only be $50 and you will have waited a significant amount of time to receive even that. Also, your customer has no incentive to pay you the amount owed because the customer knows that even if you sue him and take him all the way to a trial he will end up paying you no more than the $500 he was originally obligated to pay. If, on the other hand, you have a written agreement providing for the collection of attorneys' fees in the event of a lawsuit, your customer will have an incentive to pay you promptly or risk paying you substantially more and, in the event one must go all the way through a trial, you will be able to collect the amount of your dept, plus the amount you had to pay an attorney to collect it. Fourth, the agreement should make provision for the accruing of interest for late payments. The rationale behind this is similar to the rationale behind the attorneys' fees. Absent an agreement to pay interest on unpaid bills, you will probably be unable to collect interest. In addition, one would want to collect a maximum amount of interest allowed by the jurisdiction in which your business is located. The same incentive discussed earlier is provided and at least you will receive payment for the use of your money, something that every professional lender absolutely requires. This is especially significant if you have borrowed money to finance your business and are paying an interest rate to the bank for the use of their funds. It is only fair that people who use your funds, in this case against your will, pay for the privilege.

Summary

The scope of government involvement in small business is wide and far-reaching. This chapter does not attempt to give you a broad overview of every legal aspect of owning a small business. It is hoped that by introducing the various forms of doing business and highlighting some of the important everyday legal involvements the new business owner can avoid mishaps, pick the most appropriate and flexible form within which to conduct business, and keep legal expenses to a relative minimum so that the business owner can go about the business of performing the profession with some element of economic success. Owning a business, regardless of the subject matter of the business, does involve keeping up on changes and government laws and regulations, knowledge of relevant tax requirements, and the development of a basic business sense of the payment of bills and the collection of money. Eventually this business sense becomes intuitive; at the outset it is helpful to have a guide map to the basic signpost down the road of business success.

9

Evaluating Economic Opportunities

Frank E. Norton

The health services field has been a developing one in the variety of services offered, a trend that is certain to continue. Professionals in the health care field are in a good position to see new opportunities and to take advantage of them. Although ideas are the strategic element in moving into a new activity, it is important to evaluate each prospective opportunity in terms of its economic feasibility. The principal purpose of this chapter is to suggest ways to evaluate an opportunity.

To stimulate thinking about entrepreneurial opportunities in the health care field, I will first briefly review some of the major influences on the demand for health services, making an economic analysis of the role of population, income, price, preferences, and quality variables on the demand for health services. In the process, I will present selected empirical evidence and a discussion of health care expenditures and their financing.

The second part of this chapter is devoted to how pro forma income statements may be formulated for a prospective business opportunity and used to evaluate such an opportunity. To illustrate the procedure a hypothetical case study is presented.

Overall Influences on the Demand for Health Services

The health services purchased by the population of the United States in any one year are the result of many variables. Nevertheless, economic analysis demonstrates that certain strategic variables are the primary influence on the demand for services, and other variables become insignificant by comparison. In this section I will discuss these strategic variables in the light of selected empirical evidence, showing the role they have played and are likely to play with respect to health service purchases.

Demographic Trends

The demand for health services is fundamentally based on the size and age distribution of the population. Table 9-1 provides information on these aspects of the United States population. Population estimates and projections are provided from 1950 through the turn of the century.[1] The table shows that the percentage rate of growth of the population has been declining since 1950 and that it is expected to continue to decline as the year 2000 approaches, although the overall number of people will increase. However, a slight increase in the percentage rate of growth is expected from 1980 to 1990, followed by a further decline. Calculations derived from the table data indicate that these statements also hold true for absolute rate of growth. These results are due to the post-World War II baby boom. The growth rate of the population at any given time is dependent on the difference between births and deaths plus net immigration. The birth rate tends to vary more than the death rate, the latter showing a slow downward trend in peacetime. Until very recently, net immigration has not changed very much. Thus changes in the growth rate of the population tend to be dominated by changes in the birth rate. The large number of women born in the 1950s are now in their prime childbearing years, and this will produce an *echo effect* in the birth rate in the next ten years. This is shown dramatically by the percentage change in the number of persons under five years of age, which increased 13.1 percent in the period 1950-1955 and will increase 17.4 percent in the period 1980-1985. Consequently, the maturation of members of the postwar baby boom will increase the rate of growth of the population in the next decade.

[1] These are Series II projections. The lower Series I and higher Series III projections are based on less likely assumptions.

It is clear that the population as a whole will be older. The median age will increase from the current value of 30.2 years to 35.5 in the year 2000. The demand for health services is higher for the older age-groups than for the younger. An examination of Table 9-1 shows that the share of the population in the older age-groups tends to rise in most instances as the turn of the century approaches. Of special significance is the increase in the proportion of the population in the 65 years and over category. This group represented 8.1 percent of the population in 1950 and 9.8 percent in 1970, and is expected to represent 12.2 percent in both 1990 and 2000. Demographic trends suggest that the potential demand for health services will be increasing at a slower rate as we approach the year 2000, particularly after 1990. The shift in the age distribution toward older people will tend to ameliorate this basic tendency somewhat.

Although demographic trends influence the *potential* demand for health services, we are ultimately concerned with the *effective* demand for health services, which takes into account the ability of individuals to finance health expenditures. For the moment we are concerned only with those health expenditures financed by private sources.

Income and Price Trends

Income and the relative price of health services have an important influence on the demand for health services. Table 9-2 presents information on real per capita disposable income for the period 1950-1990, as well as real per capita national health expenditures (including money spent on health-related research and construction, health services and supplies), the price of medical care, and all consumer prices for the period 1950-1975 in the United Stat s. Here disposable income is personal income less taxes, and real means that money income is adjusted for price change, that is inflation. Not only will the potential demand for health services be enhanced by the fact that there will be more people in the future and that the population will be older, but a higher standard of living will make it possible for a larger quantity of health services to be purchased per person. Real per capita disposable income is projected to increase from $4025 in 1975 to $5439 in 1990. Notwithstanding other influences, we would expect a substantial increase in real health expenditures per capita with such an increase in real per capita disposable income. The increase in real per capita health expenditures from $202 in 1950 to $475 in 1975 was due in part to the real per capita disposable

Table 9-1 Estimates and Projections of the United States

Subject	Total, all ages	Under 5 years	5 to 13 years	14 to 17 years	18 to 24 years	25 to 34 years	35 to 44 years	45 to 54 years	55 to 64 years	65 years and over	Median age
Estimates											
Population											
1950	152,271	16,410	22,423	8,444	16,075	24,036	21,637	17,453	13,396	12,397	30.2
1955	165,931	18,566	27,925	9,247	14,968	24,283	22,912	18,885	14,622	14,525	30.2
1960	180,671	20,341	32,965	11,219	16,128	22,919	24,221	20,578	15,625	16,675	29.4
1965	194,303	19,824	35,754	14,153	20,293	22,465	24,447	21,839	17,077	18,451	28.1
1970	204,878	17,148	36,636	15,910	24,687	25,294	23,142	23,310	18,664	20,087	27.9
1975	213,540	15,882	33,440	16,934	27,604	30,918	22,815	23,768	19,774	22,405	28.8
1976	215,118	15,339	32,955	16,897	28,166	32,044	23,076	23,643	20,064	22,934	29.0
Percent distribution											
1950	100.0	10.8	14.7	5.5	10.6	15.8	14.2	11.5	8.8	8.1	
1955	100.0	11.2	16.8	5.6	9.0	14.6	13.8	11.4	8.8	8.8	
1960	100.0	11.3	18.2	6.2	8.9	12.7	13.4	11.4	8.6	9.2	
1965	100.0	10.2	18.4	7.3	10.4	11.6	12.6	11.2	8.8	9.5	
1970	100.0	8.4	17.9	7.8	12.0	12.3	11.3	11.4	9.1	9.8	
1975	100.0	7.4	15.7	7.9	12.9	14.5	10.7	11.1	9.3	10.5	
1976	100.0	7.1	15.3	7.9	13.1	14.9	10.7	11.0	9.3	10.7	
Percent change											
1950-1955	+9.0	+13.1	+24.5	+9.5	-6.9	+1.0	+5.9	+8.2	+9.2	+17.2	
1955-1960	+8.9	+9.6	+18.0	+21.3	+7.7	-5.6	+5.7	+9.0	+6.9	+14.8	
1960-1965	+7.5	-2.5	+8.5	+26.2	+25.8	-2.0	+0.9	+6.1	+9.3	+10.7	
1965-1970	+5.4	-13.5	+2.5	+12.4	+21.7	+12.6	-5.3	+6.7	+9.3	+8.9	
1970-1975	+4.2	-7.4	-8.7	+6.4	+11.8	+22.2	-1.4	+2.0	+5.9	+11.5	

Projections (Series II)

Population

1980	222,159	16,020	30,197	15,763	29,462	36,172	25,721	22,698	21,198	24,927	30.2
1985	232,880	18,803	29,098	14,392	27,853	39,859	31,376	22,457	21,737	27,305	31.5
1990	243,513	19,437	32,568	12,771	25,148	41,086	36,592	25,311	20,776	29,824	32.8
1995	252,750	18,775	35,392	14,226	23,222	38,154	40,178	30,810	20,592	31,401	34.2
2000	260,378	17,852	35,080	16,045	24,653	34,450	41,344	35,875	23,257	31,822	35.5

Percent distribution

1980	100.0	7.2	13.6	7.1	13.3	16.3	11.6	10.2	9.5	11.2
1985	100.0	8.1	12.5	6.2	12.0	17.1	13.5	9.6	9.3	11.7
1990	100.0	8.0	13.4	5.2	10.3	16.9	15.0	10.4	8.5	12.2
1995	100.0	7.4	14.0	5.6	9.2	15.1	15.9	12.2	8.1	12.4
2000	100.0	6.9	13.5	6.2	9.5	13.2	15.9	13.8	8.9	12.2

Percent change

1975-1980	+4.0	+0.9	-9.7	-6.9	+6.7	+17.0	+12.7	-4.5	+7.2	+11.3
1980-1985	+4.8	+17.4	-3.6	-8.7	-5.5	+10.2	+22.0	-1.1	+2.5	+9.5
1985-1990	+4.6	+3.4	+11.9	-11.3	-9.7	+3.1	+16.6	+12.7	-4.4	+9.2
1990-1995	+3.8	-3.4	+8.7	+11.4	-7.7	-7.1	+9.8	+21.7	-0.9	+5.3
1995-2000	+3.0	-4.9	-0.9	+12.8	+6.2	-9.7	+2.9	+16.4	+12.9	+1.3

Source: *Current Population Reports*, Series P-25, No. 310, tables 1, 2, 5; No. 519, table 1; No. 614, table 1; No. 643, table 1.

[a] Populations in thousands. As of July 1. Includes armed forces overseas. Figures inside heavy lines for population and percent change represent in whole or in part the survivors of projected births.

income. (There is approximately a linear relationship between such expenditures and income.)

The demand for health services, like that of other goods and services, is influenced by the relative price of health services compared to all other goods and services. In general, if the price of a service increases relative to that of other goods and services that are to some extent substitutes, the quantity demanded of the service will decrease, other things being equal. Table 9-2 shows that since 1967, the base year, medical care prices have risen 61.2 percent for the same period. This suggests that the volume of health services would have increased somewhat more than they did if the price increase for health services had been the same as that for all other consumer goods and services. The greater price increase for medical care tempered the increase in the amount demanded of such services. However, because of the rapid and extensive development of health insurance, this influence has been limited.

Table 9.2   United States Per Capita Real Disposable Income, Per Capita Real National Health Expenditures, and Indexes of Medical Care and All Consumer Prices

Year	Per capita real disposable income, 1972 dollars	Per capita real national health expenditures, 1972 dollars	Medical care prices 1967 = 100	All consumer prices 1967 = 100
1950	$ 2386	$ 202	53.7	72.1
1955	2577	216	64.8	80.2
1960	2697	245	79.1	88.7
1965	3152	322	89.5	94.5
1970	3619	394	120.6	116.3
1975	4025	475	168.6	161.2
1980	4458			
1985	4866			
1990	5439			

Sources: *Economic Report of the President,* January 1980, (Washington: Government Printing Office, 1980) for Real Disposable Income, 1950-1974; Consumer Price Indexes; Population. *The UCLA National Business Forecast,* Long-Term Forecast 1980-1990 for Real Disposable Income, 1980-1990. R.M. Gibson, "National Health Expenditures, 1978," *Health Care Financing Review,* (1):1-36, Summer 1979; Office of Research, Demonstrations, and Statistics, Health Care Financing Administration for National Health Expenditures. Per Capita Real National Health Expenditures calculated on basis of data from above sources.

In summary, income and price trends have influenced the demand for health services quite apart from demographic trends. Income has had a positive effect, whereas price probably has had a negative effect. What the future will bring is uncertain. Real per capita income will be much higher in 1990 but the prospective movement of medical care prices versus all other prices is not clear. The UCLA long-term forecast projects an increase in all consumer prices of 118 percent between 1980 and 1990.

Changing Preferences and Quality of Health Care

In recent years, the population has become much more health conscious and this trend is certain to continue. It is likely, for example, that much more attention will be given to preventive medicine. Individuals will probably take increasing responsibility for their own health with the help of health care professionals. These circumstances have increased the demand for health services quite independently of the variables just discussed. Furthermore, the quality of health services has improved. Technological advances in health care involving sophisticated treatment processes such as intensive care units, radiation therapy, and renal dialysis have become fairly common. These advances usually involve more highly skilled medical personnel. Therefore, the advances in the quality of health care have led to a further increase in the demand for health services because people now value such services more highly.

Thus the rise in the demand for health services is also significantly related to changing preferences and quality of health care.

Health Care Expenditures and Their Financing

The aforementioned influences on the demand for health services are reflected in total health expenditures. These expenditures are the product of the quantities of the various health services multiplied by the price of each service. Table 9-3 provides information on United States national health expenditures for selected years between 1929 and 1978. National health expenditures include the amount spent for all health services and supplies and health-related research and construction in the United States during a given period. It should be noted that these expenditure totals are not adjusted for the inflation in health care prices, as were those in Table 9-2. The table shows that per capita expenditures for 1978 were more than ten times the level of 1950, increasing from $82 to $863 per person. Private expenditures are outlays for services provided or paid for by nongovern-

Table 9-3 National Health Expenditures, According to Source of Funds: United States, Selected Years 1929-1978[a]

Year	All health expenditures in billions	Private			Public		
		Amount in billions	Amount per capita	Percentage of total	Amount in billions	Amount per capita	Percentage of total
1929	$ 3.6	$ 3.2	$ 25.49	86.4	$ 0.5	$ 4.00	13.6
1935	2.9	2.4	18.30	80.8	0.6	4.34	19.2
1940	4.0	3.2	23.61	79.7	0.8	6.03	20.3
1950	12.7	9.2	59.62	72.8	3.4	22.24	27.2
1955	17.7	13.2	78.33	74.3	4.6	27.05	25.7
1960	26.9	20.3	110.20	75.3	6.6	36.10	24.7
1965	43.0	32.3	163.29	75.1	10.7	54.13	24.9
1966	47.3	34.0	169.81	71.8	13.3	66.71	28.2
1967	52.7	33.9	167.61	64.4	18.8	97.74	35.6
1968	58.9	37.1	181.40	63.0	21.8	106.76	37.0
1969	66.2	41.6	201.83	62.9	24.5	118.87	37.1
1970	74.7	47.5	227.71	63.5	27.3	130.93	36.5
1971	82.8	51.4	244.12	62.1	31.4	148.97	37.9
1972	92.7	57.7	271.78	62.3	35.0	164.69	37.7
1973	102.3	63.6	297.17	62.1	38.8	181.22	37.9
1974	115.6	69.0	319.99	59.7	46.6	216.00	40.3
1975	131.5	75.8	348.61	57.7	55.7	255.96	42.3
1976	148.9	86.6	394.73	58.2	62.3	284.06	41.8
1977	170.0	100.7	455.27	59.2	69.3	313.50	40.8
1978[b]	192.4	114.3	512.62	59.4	78.1	350.40	40.6

Sources: R.M. Gibson, "National Health Expenditures, 1978," *Health Care Financing Review* 1(1):1-36, Summer 1979. Office of Research, Demonstrations, and Statistics, Health Care Financing Administration: Selected data.
[a] Data are compiled by the Health Care Financing Administration.

ment sources—consumers, insurance companies, private industry, and philanthropic organizations. Public expenditures are outlays for services provided or paid for by federal, state, and local government agencies or expenditures required by governmental action. They include Medicare and Medicaid; programs that provide services directly to such groups as veterans, members of the armed services, and crippled children, as well as worker's compensation benefits. Note that although per capita private expenditures were $513 in 1978 as compared to $350 for per capita public expenditures, the share of the latter in total expenditures has been growing rapidly, especially since the mid-1960s.

Table 9-4 breaks down national health expenditures into those for health services and supplies on the one hand, and those for research and construction on the other, on a percentage basis. The former category is broken down by detailed services and supplies. Since 1950, hospital care and nursing home care have taken a larger share of total expenditures for services and supplies, and physicians' services, drugs, and drug sundries have taken a smaller share. It is not clear from the data available how these shifts in expenditures are dependent on varying price movements. Certainly the shifts do not reflect entirely a change in the volume of services rendered.

The last point is illustrated in Table 9-5, where information is provided on personal health care expenditures and factors affecting their growth for the period 1969-1978. Personal health care expenditures are outlays for goods and services relating directly to patient care—that is, total national health expenditures minus expenditures for research and construction, expenses for administering health insurance programs, and government public health activities. The table shows that the increase in prices was responsible for the largest proportion of the increase in personal health care expenditures, except for the years 1972 and 1973 when the Economic Stabilization Program involving wage and price controls was in effect. Over the entire 1969-1978 period, price increases accounted for 63 percent of the increases in expenditures.

Population was responsible for 7 percent of the growth in expenditures, whereas intensity accounted for 30 percent for the period 1969-1978. Intensity reflects changes in the use or kinds of services and supplies and is a rubric for the influence of changes in income, preferences, and health service quality discussed previously.

Perhaps one of the greatest changes in the health services field has been in the financing of health expenditures through third-party payments, as is clear from Table 9-6. Third-party payments are those made by parties other than the consumer. The table shows that direct payments have fallen from 52 percent in the mid-1960s to 30 percent in 1977 of total personal health care expenditures. The decline has been even more dramatic in the case of persons 65 years of age and over.

Table 9-4 National Health Expenditures and Percent Distribution, According to Type of Expenditure: United States, Selected Years 1950-1978 [a]

Type of expenditure	Year						
	1950	1960	1965	1970	1975	1977	1978[b]
	Amount in billions						
Total	$12.7	$26.9	$43.0	$74.7	$131.5	$170.0	$192.4
	Percent distribution						
All expenditures	100.0	100.0	100.0	100.0	100.0	100.0	100.0
Health services and supplies	92.4	93.6	92.0	92.9	93.7	94.9	95.1
Hospital Care	30.4	33.8	32.4	37.2	39.7	40.0	39.5
Physician services	21.7	21.1	19.7	19.2	19.0	18.4	18.3
Dentist services	7.6	7.4	6.5	6.4	6.3	6.9	6.9
Nursing home care	1.5	2.0	4.8	6.3	7.5	7.9	8.2
Other professional services	3.1	3.2	2.4	2.1	2.0	2.2	2.2
Drugs and drug sundries	13.6	13.6	13.4	11.3	9.0	8.1	7.9
Eyeglasses and appliances	3.9	2.9	4.3	2.8	2.3	2.0	2.0
Expenses for prepayment	3.6	4.1	3.4	3.1	2.8	4.6	5.2
Government public health activities	2.9	1.5	1.9	1.9	2.4	2.5	2.6
Other health services	4.2	4.1	3.0	2.8	2.8	2.4	2.3
Research and construction	7.6	6.4	8.1	7.1	6.3	5.2	4.9
Research	0.9	2.5	3.4	2.5	2.4	2.2	2.2
Construction	6.7	3.9	4.7	4.6	3.9	3.0	2.7

Sources: R.M. Gibson, "National Health Expenditures, 1978," *Health Care Financing Review* 1(1):1-36, Summer 1979. Office of Research, Demonstrations, and Statistics, Health Care Financing Administration: Selected data.

[a] Data are compiled by the Health Care Financing Administration.
[b] Preliminary estimates.

Table 9-5 Personal Health Care Expenditures, Average Annual Percent Change, and Percent Distribution of Factors Affecting Growth: United States, 1969-1978. [a]

Year	Personal health care expenditures in millions	Average annual percent change [b]	Factors affecting growth (percent distribution)			
			All factors	Prices	Population	Intensity [c]
1969-1978		12.6	100.0	63.0	7.0	30.0
1969	$ 57,888	—	—	—	—	—
1970	65,723	13.5	100.0	54.0	8.0	38.0
1971	72,115	9.7	100.0	65.0	11.0	24.0
1972	79,870	10.8	100.0	42.0	8.0	50.0
1973	88,471	10.8	100.0	43.0	7.0	50.0
1974	100,885	14.0	100.0	71.0	6.0	23.0
1975	116,297	15.3	100.0	80.0	5.0	15.0
1976	132,127	13.6	100.0	71.0	7.0	22.0
1977	149,139	12.9	100.0	68.0	7.0	25.0
1978	167,911	12.6	100.0	68.0	7.0	25.0

Sources: R.M. Gibson, "National Health Expenditures, 1978," *Health Care Financing Review* 1(1):1-36, Summer 1979. Office of Research, Demonstrations, and Statistics, Health Care Financing Administration: Selected data.

 [a] Data are compiled by the Health Care Financing Administration.
 [b] Refers to one year periods unless otherwise noted.
 [c] Represents changes in use and/or kinds of service and supplies.

Table 9.6   Personal Health Care Per Capita Expenditures and Percent Distribution, According to Source of Payment and Age: United States, Fiscal Years 1966-1967 [a]

Age and Year	All personal health care expenditures	All sources	Direct payment	Source of Payment (percent distribution)				
				Total	Third-party payment			
					Private Health insurance	Philanthropy and industry	Government
All ages							
1966	$ 181.96	100.0	51.5	48.5	24.7	2.0	21.8
1967	205.45	100.0	45.4	54.6	22.6	1.8	30.1
1968	228.75	100.0	41.1	58.9	22.4	1.7	34.8
1969	256.59	100.0	39.8	60.2	23.2	1.6	35.5
1970	289.76	100.0	40.4	59.6	24.0	1.5	34.2
1971	320.84	100.0	39.1	60.9	24.9	1.4	34.6
1972	353.00	100.0	37.6	62.4	24.9	1.4	36.1
1973	386.84	100.0	36.8	63.2	25.4	1.4	36.4
1974 [b]	425.15	100.0	36.1	63.9	25.2	1.3	37.3
1975 [b]	488.23	100.0	33.6	66.4	25.4	1.3	39.7
1976 [a,b]	551.50	100.0	32.5	67.5	26.0	1.3	40.2
1977 [c,d]	646.11	100.0	30.3	69.7	27.6	2.0	40.1
Under 65 years							
1966	154.96	100.0	51.1	48.9	27.3	2.2	19.4
1967	171.55	100.0	48.1	51.9	28.0	2.2	21.7
1968	185.39	100.0	46.0	54.0	28.6	2.0	23.3
1969	206.36	100.0	44.2	55.8	29.8	1.9	24.1

1970	232.50	100.0	43.3	56.7	31.0	1.9	23.9
1971	255.09	100.0	41.1	58.9	32.6	1.8	24.5
1972	278.23	100.0	38.4	61.6	33.0	1.5	26.8
1973	309.45	100.0	38.3	61.7	33.2	1.7	26.8
1974 [b]	347.87	100.0	39.0	61.0	32.3	1.7	27.0
1975 [b]	390.79	100.0	36.5	63.5	33.3	1.6	28.6
1976 [c,d]	437.83	100.0	34.9	65.1	34.5	1.7	29.0
1977 [c,d]	514.25	100.0	31.9	68.1	36.4	2.6	29.1
65 years and over							
1966	445.25	100.0	53.2	46.8	15.9	1.1	29.8
1967	535.03	100.0	37.0	63.0	5.9	0.8	56.4
1968	646.65	100.0	27.5	72.5	5.3	0.6	66.6
1969	735.19	100.0	28.0	72.0	5.4	0.5	66.1
1970	828.31	100.0	32.6	67.4	5.5	0.5	61.4
1971	925.98	100.0	34.2	65.8	5.4	0.5	60.0
1972	1,033.51	100.0	35.5	64.5	5.2	0.4	58.9
1973	1,081.35	100.0	33.0	67.0	5.4	0.4	61.1
1974 [b]	1,109.54	100.0	28.0	72.0	5.7	0.5	65.9
1975 [b]	1,335.72	100.0	26.3	73.7	5.4	0.4	68.0
1976 [c]	1,521.36	100.0	26.5	73.5	5.4	0.4	67.7
1977 [c,d]	1,745.17	100.0	26.5	73.5	5.8	0.7	67.0

[a] Data are compiled by the Health Care Financing Administration.
[b] Revised estimates.
[c] Preliminary estimates.
[d] Data for fiscal year ending September 30; all other data for fiscal year ending June 30.
Sources: Gibson, R. M., and M. S. Mueller, "Age differences in Health Care Spending, Fiscal Year 1974," *Social Security Bulletin* 38(6):3-14, June 1975. R. M. Gibson, M. S. Mueller, and C. R. Fisher, "Age Differences in Health Care Spending, Fiscal Year 1976, *Social Security Bulletin* 40(8):3-14, August, 1977. R. M. Gibson and C. R. Fisher, "Age Differences in Health Care Spending, Fiscal Year 1977," *Social Security Bulletin* 42(1):3-16, January 1979.

Another fact shown by Table 9-6 is the much larger per capita personal health care expenditures for persons 65 years and over compared to those under 65 years. For the under-65 age-group, per capita expenditures rose from $155 in 1966 to $514 in 1977. Per capita expenditures for the over-65 age-group rose from $445 in 1966 to $1745 in 1977. As of 1977, expenditures for the latter group were 3.4 times that for the former group, which supports our earlier emphasis on age distribution as a determinant of the demand for health services. Also, the table indicates the importance of government in financing health services for the elderly, namely such programs as Medicare and Medicaid.

Pro Forma Income Statements

The most important task for a health care professional who wishes to become an entrepreneur is to develop an economically feasible idea. Ask yourself what you are capable of doing for which there is likely to be a significant market. Usually individuals who have been in the health care field for a few years will have a number of ideas. The purpose of the first section of this chapter was to help stimulate thinking about potential activities that might be undertaken. Earlier chapters provide examples of what other entrepreneurs have done.

An economic analysis of various ideas or potential activities will show that they involve different degrees of *profitability* and *risk*. What we want to know is which of these potential activities are economically feasible. My purpose here is to outline a procedure for *quantifying* the profitability of alternative potential activities. This procedure can be used for testing the economic feasibility of a project before it is actually undertaken.

The Nature of an Income Statement

The central concept in quantitatively evaluating alternative economic opportunities is that of the business income statement. Basically the traditional income statement is a summary of the results of business operations over an *interval of time*. It deals with the flow of business activity as it occurred between two points in time as reflected in *revenues* and *costs* and consequently *profits or net income*. The income statements with which most people are familiar are prepared by accountants and are essentially backward-looking, because they are prepared from historical data. However, the version of the income statement that we are concerned with is *forward-looking*. It deals with forecasts or projections of revenues and costs and thus expected profits or expected net income.[2] Such a statement is called a *pro forma income statement*. In short, such a statement reflects the plans for business operation for a future interval of time, such as a month, a quarter, a year, or perhaps several years. Underlying it will be various budgets, such as the sales budget and the production budget with a statement of costs and attendant requirements depending upon the nature of the business involved. Ultimately, since profits are the key to the survival of a business undertaking, the pro forma, income statement focuses on how business decisions will influence profits through revenues and costs for a future period. It provides an evaluation of the prospective overall performance of the business undertaking.

Pro forma income statements are not only useful in assessing the economic feasibility of a business opportunity but are typically required by lenders such as banks as part of the information called for in loan applications. Moreover, they represent what is essentially a business plan against which realized results may be compared; that is, they may be used for control purposes.

Table 9-7 is a pro forma income statement for the hypothetical case study described in the next section. In subsequent sections I will give a general economic analysis of the variables influencing such projections or forecasts in a pro forma income statement. This is done because different economic opportunities involve somewhat different approaches to the making of the forecasts. I will also explain how the figures in Table 9-7 were derived on the basis of information from the hypothetical case study.

A Hypothetical Case Study

A nurse has been practising her profession for seven years. She is employed in a hospital at $1600 per month. For the last five years she has wanted to become a dietary consultant and has taken a number of courses on diet, and she has written a short book on diet and health. To date she has hesitated to open a private practice as a dietary consultant because there is so much information available on

---

[2] Income statements are formulated on an accrual basis rather than a cash basis. All revenue is included when earned even though payment is received later and all costs are deducted as soon as incurred even though they may be paid for later.

diet in the form of books and various programs. In the last six months, however, she has developed a new idea on how a diet program should be approached and now she believes she would like to open a private practice.

In her view, though there are many diets that meet formal dietary criteria, most people do not stay on them in the long run because they are not very palatable. She believes that if people could have

Table 9-7 Pro Forma Income Statement

| | Quarter | | | | |
	I	II	III	IV	Year
Revenues					
Professional services	$ 6,000	7,500	9,000	10,500	$33,000
Vitamins	1,680	2,100	2,520	2,940	9,240
Computer diet	3,000	4,500	6,000	7,500	21,000
Total revenues	10,680	14,100	17,520	20,940	63,240
Cost of goods sold					
Books	$ 576	720	864	1,008	$ 3,168
Vitamins	672	840	1,008	1,176	3,696
Computer diet	1,362	1,947	2,532	3,117	8,958
Total cost of goods sold	2,610	3,507	4,404	5,301	15,822
Gross profit	$ 8,070	10,593	13,116	15,639	$47,418
Operating costs					
Office supplies	$ 60				$ 60
Advertising	2,000	1,500	1,000	1,000	5,500
Professional services	550	150	150	150	1,000
Rent	3,000	3,000	3,000	3,000	12,000
Telephone	150	120	120	120	510
Utilities	75	75	75	75	300
Insurance	1,200				1,200
Depreciation	65	65	65	65	260
Taxes	101	126	151	176	554
Total operating costs	7,201	5,036	4,561	4,586	21,384
Net profits	$ 869	5,557	8,555	11,053	$ 26,034

diets that permitted at least some of the foods that they liked, they would be more likely to stay on the diet. Her approach was to make a list of all major foods classified by category, then to ask each patient to rank them in order of preference. Then she formulated a custom diet that maximized the foods preferred subject to dietary constraints relating to the health status of the individual. Her mathematical training as a university undergraduate suggested that this was a determinate optimization problem. Therefore she hired an applied mathematician who was also a computer programmer and asked him to solve the optimization problem mathematically using her approach and to write a computer program for its implementation. He was paid $500.

She envisages undertaking two related activities. First, she would like to advertise the computer diet in newspapers. Persons who respond to such advertisements would be sent a three-page questionnaire on which they would indicate relevant medical history and rank all foods in terms of preference. Upon her receipt of the questionnaire, the optimal diet—taking into account both food preferences and dietary constraints—would be calculated and returned. The charge would be $25. A computer service firm has agreed to perform these calculations for $7 including return mailing. Second, she wants to open an office to practice as a dietary consultant. In this practice she would provide a *diet package* consisting of a diagnostic examination and consultation, a copy of her diet and health book, and the computer diet, for a fee of $125. Laboratory tests would be performed by a laboratory and the patient would be billed separately. She would also sell a packet of vitamins, if the patient desired to purchase them, for $35. Follow-up consultation would be at a fee of $40.

The Projection of Revenues

Revenues are the product of the quantities of the goods or services purchased multiplied by the price of (or fee for) the services. There may be a number of types of goods or services provided, in which case revenues for the business undertaking are simply the summation of the revenues derived from the separate goods or services. The amount of a good or service demanded depends on a host of variables that are unique to the goods or services in question. Nevertheless, there are certain strategic variables that tend to dominate the demand for a good or service and are almost always of significance. Some of these have been mentioned earlier in connection with the review of overall influences on the demand for health services. These are the most important: price of the good or service, price of close substitute goods or services, income, advertising, quality of the good or service, preferences, and population. Of these variables, the seller frequently has control over three of them, which are termed *policy variables:* the *price* of the good or service, *advertising,* and the *quality* of the good or service. These are variables the entrepreneurial decision maker can manipulate with the objective of changing the amount demanded, and ultimately profits or net income. Presumably the decision maker aims at a set of values for these variables that will maximize profits.

The amount demanded varies inversely with the price, other things being equal. Some goods or services are quite sensitive to price changes, whereas others are not. This sensitivity will tend to be high where close substitutes (or competition) for the good or service exist and where a large proportion of income is spent on the good or service and vice versa. Sensitivity will also be related to preference and income differentials in the population.

In a similar manner, the amount demanded varies directly with both advertising and quality of good or service, other things being equal. Again the sensitivity varies among goods or services. These two variables also influence cost as well as the amount demanded and revenues.

Consequently price, advertising, and quality policies will influence the amount demanded of a good or service and thereby revenues. The implementation of these decisions must be assessed as best as possible.

External environmental variables are also important in forecasting the amount demanded of a good or service. The amount demanded varies directly with the price of close substitutes (or competitors' prices), other things being equal. Another important variable is income, to which the amount demanded of most goods or services is positively related. Changes in general and regional business conditions are reflected in this variable and thus affect demand. Finally, the amount demanded is usually positively related to both preferences and population. The impact of these variables has been discussed earlier.

I turn now to a brief explanation of how the revenue projections in Table 9-7 were developed. The roman numerals stand for the quarter of the year involved; that is, I represents the first quarter, and so on.

Revenues
Professional services (diet package)

I.	($125) (4 patients) (4 wks.) (3 mo.) =	$ 6,000
II.	($125) (5 patients) (4 wks.) (3 mo.) =	7,500
III.	($125) (6 patients) (4 wks.) (3 mo.) =	9,000
IV.	($125) (7 patients) (4 wks.) (3 mo.) =	10,500
	Total for year	$33,000

Vitamins

I.	($ 35) (48 patients)	= $ 1,680
II.	($ 35) (60 patients)	= 2,100
III.	($35) (72 patients)	= 2,520
IV.	($ 35) (84 patients)	= 2,940
	Total for year	$ 9,240

Computer diet

I.	($ 25) (10 questionaires) (4 wks.) (3 mo.) = $	3,000
II.	($ 25) (15 questionaires) (4 wks.) (3 mo.) =	4,500
III.	($ 25) (20 questionaires) (4 wks.) (3 mo.) =	6,000
IV.	($ 25) (25 questionaires) (4 wks.) (3 mo.) =	7,500
	Total for year	$ 21,000

The product mix consists of professional services—the diet package including diagnostic examination and consultation, diet and health book, and computer diet—the vitamins for sale, and the computer diet, which is also sold by mail. The professional services are conducted in a modern office building located in a suburban trading and business area having adequate parking and convenient freeway access. The economic base of the area is growing in population, particularly in the 25-45 age-group of middle to upper-income persons, most of whom are well educated and reside nearby. Business activity is likely to continue to expand in the area at a rapid rate, at least for the next half-decade. The Yellow Pages of the telephone directory indicate only a few existing competitors. It is believed that the diet package is unique, and that the estimated number of patients should be forthcoming at a fee of $125, which is not out of line with that charged by competitors. To promote the private practice, the nurse plans (among other things) to give a brief university extension course on diet and health, write newspaper articles on the subject, and actively participate in community relations, all activities in keeping with her professional image.

It is thought that patients will almost always purchase the vitamins recommended as well. They are specially packaged and designed for the custom diets. The estimate assumes this to be so. The health and diet book is supplied to each patient without additional charge.

The computer diet is to be marketed through initially quite heavy advertising in the newspaper. Patients cut out the coupon provided and send it in together with $25. They are then sent a questionnaire, which they complete and return. Optimal diets are computed and returned. These patients will probably be drawn from a somewhat wider geographic area than those in the private practice. It is estimated that, after a transitory period, five questionnaires a day would be processed.

The Projection of Costs

Costs may be divided into *cost of goods sold* and *operating costs*. Where a business purchases goods and resells them to customers, the cost of goods sold is the net change in inventories from the beginning of a period to the end of a period plus the purchases during the period. These costs vary directly with sales volume or revenues. If the business manufactures a product, then these costs are also included in the cost of goods sold. The latter costs also tend to vary directly with sales volume or revenues, but whatever part does not so vary is called a *fixed cost*. Those costs that vary directly with revenues or output are called *variable costs*. Operating costs usually do not vary with sales volume or revenues and are therefore fixed costs.

Costs are important not only in their influence on profits but also in the pricing of goods and services.[3] In general, the optimal price for a good or service depends on costs, on the one hand, and the sensitivity of demand to price changes on the other.[4]

---

[3] If the product mix of a business is approximately unchanging, profits may be forecast by the equation,

$$\pi = R - FC - (VC/R) \bullet R$$

where π = profits; R = revenues; FC = fixed costs; VC = variable costs; VC/R = a constant in this analysis; no account is taken of demand—that is, how price influences the amount sold.

[4] Technically, $P^* = \dfrac{VC/q}{1 - \dfrac{1}{\eta}}$ and $\dfrac{1}{\eta} = u$ and $\eta = \dfrac{P}{q} \bullet \dfrac{\delta q}{\delta P}$

where P^* = optimal or profit-maximizing price; q = amounts sold or produced; η = direct price-elasticity of demand, u = optimal markup. (For more information, see any intermediate economics text.)

Consequently, both demand and cost play a role in the determination of the appropriate price. The following breakdown shows how the cost projections in Table 7 were made.

Costs

Cost of goods sold
    Books

Beginning inventory	($12) (48 patients) (½) =	$288
Purchases	($12) (48 patients) =	576
Less ending inventory	($12) (48 patients) (½) =	288

Inventory on hand at the beginning of a quarter is assumed to be one-half that purchased during the quarter, and ending inventories are assumed to be the same. The purchases are as follows:

I.	($12) (48 patients) =	$ 576
II.	($12) (60 patients) =	720
III.	($12) (72 patients) =	864
IV.	($12) (84 patients) =	1008
Total for year		$3,168

Vitamins

Beginning inventory	($14) (48 patients) (½) =	$ 336
Purchases	($14) (48 patients) =	672
Less ending inventory	($14) (48 patients) (½) =	336

Inventories are treated the same as for books. The purchases are as follows:

I. ($14) (48 patients) =		$ 672
II. ($14) (60 patients) =		840
III. ($14) (72 patients) =		1008
IV. ($14) (84 patients) =		1176
Total for year		$3,696

Computer diet
Questionnaire (paper and printing)

I. ($1) (48 patients) + ($1) (120 returns) =	$ 168
II. ($1) (60 patients) + ($1) (180 returns) =	240
III. ($1) (72 patients) + ($1) (240 returns) =	312
IV. ($1) (84 patients) + ($1) (300 returns) =	384
Total for year	$1,104

Postage

I. ($0.15)	(120)	=	$ 18
II. ($0.15)	(180)	=	27
III. ($0.15)	(240)	=	36
IV. ($0.15)	(300)	=	45
Total for one year			$126

Computing

I. ($7) (48 + 120) =	$1176
II. ($7) (60 + 180) =	1680
III. ($7) (72 + 240) =	2184
IV. ($7) (84 + 300) =	2688
Total for year	$7728

Then the total of all cost associated with the computer diet is:

I.	$1362
II.	1947
III.	2532
IV.	3118
Total	$8958

A publisher has agreed to produce the diet and health book for $14 a copy. Each patient in private practice receives one without extra charge.

The vitamins are produced by a pharmaceutical firm for $14. It is assumed that all patients purchase the vitamins.

The computer diet questionnaire is three pages long and produced on special paper so that the data can be read automatically as input to the computer. The cost is $1. A computer service firm will process the questionnaires using the program supplied by the nurse for $7 a questionnaire.

Operating costs

Office supplies:	Stationery with letterhead, business cards
Advertising:	Yellow Pages of the telephone directory plus newspaper
Professional services:	Accountant, $50/mo. plus $300 for setup including income tax preparation; attorney, $100
Rent:	$1000/mo. including heating, cooling and parking
Telephone:	$40/mo. plus $30 installation

Utilities: Electricity and water $25/mo.
Insurance: $1200 public liability and fixtures
Depreciation:

Item	Cost	Declining Balance (%)	Depreciation
Typewriter	$ 250	20	$ 50.00
File cabinet	75	20	15.00
Answering system	300	20	60.00
Calculator	75	20	15.00
Desk and chair	250	10	25.00
Davenport	400	10	40.00
End table	150	10	15.00
Lamps	150	10	15.00
Chairs	175	10	17.50
Pictures	75	10	7.50
	$1900		$260.00

Taxes:	Sales taxes:	
I. ($0.06) ($1680) =		$101
II. ($0.06) ($2100) =		126
III. ($0.06) ($2520) =		151
IV. ($0.06) ($2940) =		176
Total for year		$554

Implicit Revenues and Costs

The pro forma income statement based upon the projected revenues
and projected costs presented in Table 9-7 gives a forecasted profit
or net income of $26,034. This is the income upon which the federal
and state income tax would be paid. Note that no provision for the
owner's salary or return on investment has been made. The view is
often expressed that since all the profits belong to the owner there is
no point in setting up costs to represent the owner's salary and interest. S/he may withdraw the profits as s/he wishes. However, in
order to make a rational economic decision in terms of alternative
opportunities, it is necessary to allow for the salary that would be
earned in the best alternative use of one's time and for the interest
that would be earned as well if one's invested funds were used
elsewhere. These omitted costs are called *implicit opportunity interest*
and *salary* respectively. *(Opportunity costs* are the value of resources
when used in their best alternative use. *Implicit* means they are not
stated explicitly. The implicit opportunity interest rate is assumed to

be 15 percent when risk is allowed for the undertaking.) These opportunity costs are as follows:

Implicit interest, as result of investments in:
Inventory
  Books

I.	($ 576) (0.15) (1/2) (1/4) =	$ 21.60
II.	($ 720) (0.15) (1/2) (1/4) =	27.00
III.	($ 864) (0.15) (1/2) (1/4) =	32.40
IV.	($1068) (0.15) (1/2) (1/4) =	37.80

Total for year $118.80

Vitamins

I.	($ 672) (0.15) (1/2) (1/4) =	$ 12.60
II.	($ 840) (0.15) (1/2) (1/4) =	15.80
III.	($1008) (0.15) (1/2) (1/4) =	18.90
IV.	($1176) (0.15) (1/2) (1/4) =	22.10

Total for year $ 69.40

Fixtures and equipment
  ($1900) (0.15) = $ 285.00
Computer program
  ($500) (0.15) = 75.00
Implicit salary $19,200.00

The implicit interest and implicit salary are deducted from the net profit, as Table 9-8 shows:

Table 9-8 Net Profit Adjusted for Implicit Opportunity Costs

	I	II	III	IV	Total
Net Profit	$869	$5,557	$8,555	$11,053	$26,034
Implicit Interest	125	133	140	150	584
Implicit Salary	4,800	4,800	4,800	4,800	19,200
Adjusted net profit	(4,056)	624	3,615	6,103	$ 6,286

Thus, after allowing for all opportunity costs, the projected net profit is only $6286. In view of the substantial risk exposure as a result of undertaking this activity, it does not seem like a very satisfactory return. However, to the extent that the projections are probably on the conservative side and that the market potential for both the professional practice and computer diet appears very promising in the future years,[5] the project may well be worth undertaking.

Nonpecuniary Motivation

Not all owners of a business are motivated by profit alone. Some desire the independence that owning their own business provides. They may in some cases not like to work for other people, or may not be able to in the long run because of temperament. As they become older, the satisfaction of making their own decisions may be important to them. These considerations often are given some weight and thus the decision does not rest solely on expected profits or net income alone. They are concerned with their total satisfaction, rather than their pecuniary income alone.

[5] For example, no follow-up consultation has been allowed for in the present treatment; for such a service a fee of $40 would be made.

Bibliography

Bunn, V.A. *Buying and Selling a Small Business,* 2nd Ed. Small Business Administration. Washington, D.C.: US Government Printing Office, 1979.

Economic Report of the President. Transmitted to Congress, January 1980. Washington, DC: US Government Printing Office, 1980.

Gibson, R.M. "National Health Expenditure, 1978." *Health Care Financing Review* I: 1-36, Summer 1979.

Gibson, R.M., and Fisher, C.R. "Age Differences in Health Care Spending, Fiscal Year 1977." *Social Security Bulletin* 42(1): 3-16, January 1979.

Gibson, R.M., and Mueller, M.S. "Age Differences in Health Care Spending, Fiscal Year 1974." *Social Security Bulletin* 38(6): 3-14, June 1975.

Gibson, R.M.; Mueller, M.S.; and Fisher, C.R. "Age Differences in Health Care Spending, Fiscal Year 1976." *Social Security Bulletin* 40(8): 3-14, August 1977.

Koontz, H., and O'Donnell, C. *Principles of Management.* New York: McGraw-Hill, 1978.

Krentzman, H.C. *Managing for Profits.* Small Business Administration. Washington, DC: US Government Printing Office, 1968.

Metcalf, W.O. *Starting and Managing a Small Business of Your Own,* 3rd Ed. The Starting and Managing Series, vol. 1, Small Business Administration. Washington, DC: US Government Printing Office, 1973.

Shuchat, J.; Holt, N.; and Reyal, M.L. *Something Ventured, Something Gained: An Advanced Curriculum for Small Business Management.* Vol. II. Small Business Management and Ownership. US Office of Education: Department of Health, Education, and Welfare. Washington, DC: US Government Printing Office, 1979.

Small Business Administration. *Business Plan for Small Service Firms.* Small Marketers Aid No. 153, October 1973.

The UCLA National Business Forecast, Long-Term Forecast 1980-1990, October 1980. Rockville, Maryland: General Electric Information Services, 1980.

US Bureau of the Census. "Projections of the Population of the United States: 1977-2050." *Current Population Reports*, Series P-25, No. 704. Washington, DC: US Government Printing Office, 1977.

US Bureau of the Census. *Employment Projections for the 1980s.* Bulletin 2030. Washington, DC: US Government Printing Office, 1977.

US Bureau of the Census. *Statistical Abstract of the United States,* 100th ed. Washington, DC: US Government Printing Office, 1979.

US Department of Health, Education, and Welfare. *Health: United States 1979.* Public Health Service. Hyattsville, Maryland: National Center for Health Statistics, 1980.

Wollfel, C.J. *Guides for Profit Planning*, 2nd ed. Small Business Administration, Washington, DC: US Government Printing Office, 1975.

10

Marketing CE: The Bottom Line

Arleen Gordon

Marketing is an important function in continuing education in nursing. It makes a major contribution to achieving organizational objectives, and it will become even more valuable in the future as education consumerism, competition, and fiscal stringency increase.

Traditionally, nurse educators in continuing education or staff development have either had minimal involvement with marketing or have not consciously performed that role. Like many professionals and others in nonprofit, service organizations, such as churches, educational institutions, and hospitals, they have associated marketing with profit-making, commercial enterprises that sell soap, cars, or television programs.

Professional codes of ethics discouraged active solicitation of clients. Marketing is not a subject included in nursing curricula or studied in graduate programs. These attitudes and a lack of knowledge about the subject have influenced the nurse's perception of its place within the organization and her role in relation to it.

Attitudes toward advertising practices of professionals are beginning to change. Consumer demands for information essential to sound decision making, and the need to compete more aggressively for survival in a growing marketplace, are slowly influencing advertising behavior. Law offices advertise on local television. Recently, a county visiting nurse society advertised its services on the radio. In addition to listing courses, a community college advertisement actively urged individuals to enroll. The information was surrounded by eye-catching double, black lines. The American Nurses' Association, finding current and potential members with competing demands for their time and finances, has developed an active membership/marketing division. These organizations realize the importance of the marketing function.

Both profit and nonprofit organizations face marketing problems with their environments, and the same general marketing principles can be applied to both types of organizations. Though making a profit is not the primary purpose of education, there is a similarity between the customer for profit and the client for service. The lines are blurring between management practices for the different organizations.

Education in this country is indeed a big, costly business. Del Bueno (1978) estimated that a continuing education program on coronary care, including forty or more hours of classroom time, attended by thirty nurses whose salaries, registration, and per diem costs were paid by the employing hospital, would cost $9300 and 12 lost patient care hours.

Educators in staff development caught in the paradoxical tightening of funds accompanied by increased demands for educational services, those in continuing education who must be self-supporting and rely less on grants, and private providers who must at least break even to survive know that it has become absolutely necessary to adhere to cost-effective management principles. These principles include taking a more systematic approach to effective and efficient marketing activities.

In reality, providers of continuing education and staff development are involved in some marketing functions. In a study of marketing practices in extension units in ninety member institutions of the National Association of State Universities and Land-Grant Colleges, Buchanan and Barksdale (1974) found that all units were performing marketing-like activities. Some perform these functions very well. We can all think of units that seem to know clearly what service to offer and to whom, and they consistently draw participants. Others have less proficiency and could benefit from a more formal approach.

Marketing Defined

Marketing is both a management tool and an organizational orientation. It encompasses administrative and program-development aspects. It begins long before promotion and the actual selling of an offering.

> Marketing is analysis, planning, implementation, and control of carefully formulated programs designed to bring about voluntary exchanges of values with target markets for the purpose of achieving organizational objectives. It relies heavily on designing the organization's offering in terms of the target market's needs and desires, and on using effective pricing, communication, and distribution to inform, motivate, and service the markets   [Kotler 1975, p. 5].[1]

This definition is appropriate and useful to continuing education providers. We see that marketing is a management process whose purpose is to achieve organizational objectives. Unlike the shotgun approach to programming whereby a little of everything is offered in the hope that someone out there wants it, marketing results in carefully conceived offerings aimed at those specific groups most likely to produce results. Marketing is quite responsive to consumer needs and wants. The desired outcome is a voluntary exchange satisfactory to both the organization and to individuals within the target groups. To accomplish this outcome, various tools called the "marketing mix" are used (Kotler 1975, pp. 6-7). The mix, which includes a number of elements such as promotion, place, and price, will be discussed later in the chapter.

Marketing Concepts

Examining the concepts on which marketing is based provides even more rationale for its use. The three concepts are exchange, a public, and a market.

Exchange
Exchange is the major concept in marketing. It requires two parties, each having something that the other might value, such as goods, services, or money (Kotler 1975, p. 23). Exchanges occur with consumers and others in the internal and external environments of the organization.

Currently, some exchanges in continuing education are not altogether voluntary, and participants are sometimes sent by employers without understanding why they are there. This situation

---

[1] Philip Kotler, *Marketing for Nonprofit Organizations,* ©1975. Reprinted by permission of Prentice-Hall, Inc., Englewood Cliffs, New Jersey.

often results in disgruntled or confused nurses and frustrated instructors. It influences consumer satisfaction with the program and receptivity to learning, and some thought should be given to it in advance of the program.

Program development based on needs assessment flows from the concept of exchange. What is it that we have or can develop that will be of value to the other party? What will be attractive enough to motivate them to attend and be receptive to learning or to purchase a service or a product? Is it job-related skills and knowledge? Continuing education hours for relicensure? To meet and make contacts? To get away? Considerable thought and researching of needs, wants, and other factors that influence the exchange are required to answer these questions.

The Public

Organizations exist in an environment with which they interact and are interdependent (Thompson 1967, p. 13). There are internal and external environments, made up of groups called *publics*. In Kotler's words, "A public is a distinct group of people and/or organizations that have an actual or a potential interest and/or impact on an organization [1975, p. 17]." A few of the publics of a college or university-based continuing education in nursing department are the dean of the school of nursing, the administration and staff, and the faculty (internal publics); regulatory agencies, funding agents, suppliers, competitors, current and prospective students, and health care agencies (external publics).

These groups are interrelated. Legislators enact mandatory continuing education. The regulatory agency sets requirements for meeting the law, which in turn affects the demand for offerings. The demand affects the output of the provider of continuing education or staff development, or puts stress on the organization to make some decisions about delivery roles. The requirement might also affect the participant's satisfaction with the program and attitude toward the provider.

Here's what you need to know about publics from a marketing standpoint: (1) Who are the groups? (2) How do they affect each other and the organization? (3) What exchanges occur and why? (4) Which groups would you like to trade with or see as potential markets? When you answer the fourth question, you are viewing certain public as target markets.

The Market

"A market is a distinct group of people and/or organizations that have resources which they want to exchange, or might conceivably exchange, for distinct benefits," in the words of Kotler (1975, p. 22). It is only after sorting out major publics and markets, and clarifying the exchanges and underlying motivations of each, that marketing strategies are determined.

Marketing Styles

Kotler identified three styles of marketing: aggressive, minimal, and balanced. Organizations choose different styles depending on the image they wish to project and the organization's objections. Which style seems right for your organization?

Aggressive

Aggressive or hard-sell marketing is used by many business firms and sometimes by professionals when actual sales do not meet expectations. This style relies on promotion, including high-pressure selling strategies, to generate demand. Some examples are wining and dining, slick brochures, sharp pricing and discounting, bonuses, and disparaging competitors.

Minimal

Minimal or no-sell marketing is practiced by organizations that do not consciously market. They rely on product/service availability or high-quality design to sell itself. It is assumed that demand will be there. This style is seen in hospitals, universities, and many continuing education/staff-development units.

Balanced

Balanced marketing lies between the previous two extremes. It aims to blend effectively the elements of the marketing mix so that the product sells and the consumer is satisfied (Calderon 1978; Kotler 1975, pp. 7-9).

Balanced marketing is an effective style for continuing education in nursing. It incorporates the judicious consideration of both promotion and product, plus additional factors that may influence purchasing behavior.

The Marketing Mix

The marketing mix consists of factors to consider when planning a marketing strategy. Lauffer (1977) has identified five "Right Ps": product, place, price, promotion, and partners. The elements of the mix can be used as a partial checklist for program development. The marketing objective is to use these elements as effectively and efficiently as possible to move potential clients to enroll or purchase a product or service.

The following discussion elaborates on each element as it applies to continuing education in nursing, adds the elements of the "right time" and "evaluation," and incorporates many of Benner's specific points in relation to each (Benner 1977).

The Right Product

A product is the "right" one when it matches customer needs and desires. This approach follows adult learning principles and enhances the chances of a high level of consumer satisfaction. In a study of approximately 800 registered nurses in six hospitals, Curran (1977) found that variables such as job position, clinical area, and educational background influence identified learning needs and participation in continuing education activities.

To arrive at the right product requires preliminary decisions by the organization about territory and image, an analysis of the size and demographic characteristics of the nursing population in that defined territory, and an examination of conditions that might affect market potential, such as legislation, new technology, and economic conditions.

The next step is needs assessment, (which may alternatively be conducted along with some of the above information). Interviews, performance observations, mail surveys, assessment of professional trends, and input from advisory committees can be used. Information obtained from a variety of methods and people results in a more accurate picture, but this approach is not foolproof. We are still grappling methodologically and logistically with how to target programming and levels of information for nurses from many different educational and experiential backgrounds. However, by using the results of needs assessment, a provider is much more likely to hit the mark, to produce satisfaction, and to be of service to the profession. Programs based only on a philosophy and a desired image may end up without a market.

Responsiveness to consumer needs does not mean providing

everything for everyone, but providing the right product often enough to get new customers and keep old ones. It means weighing information and providing what is feasible. It may involve assigning prerequisites for classes. Being responsive also requires taking the opportunity and the professional judgment to assume leadership in trying new delivery modes and presenting new information needed by nurses in these complex times.

The Right Place
Should an offering be held on campus? In the hospital? In a recreational setting? To determine the right place, the nature of the program, the desired or expected audience, and the image wanted need to be considered. If the program objectives can be achieved only with participants in constant attendance, then it is probably best not to hold it at a resort with beaches and competing attractions.

The Right Time
To determine the best time to offer the service, check experience related to days of the week, time of day, best months, and best seasons. Seasons are especially important to consider for single-event offerings. A large conference might not be scheduled during certain winter months if heavy snows are anticipated and travel might be difficult. Last, determine competitive events by looking, among other places, in the World Convention Dictionary; and stay clear of those dates unless the events are educationally noncompetitive.

The Right Price
The right price is a fee satisfactory to both the nurse consumer and the continuing education department. In health care settings, this may also be the "right price" for the patient. Money is not the only factor; for instance, being unable to spend time at other activities may be too high a price to pay for any benefits perceived from attending the offering. This discussion, however, will address only monetary issues.

Price is heavily dependent on what the market will allow. Sometimes this is a great deal as with well-attended management workshops priced at $300 or more. In other instances, it is not as much. When workshops were cosponsored with a number of universities in different states a few years ago, the final standard price took into consideration those states in which the local unit's experience and previous policies appeared to preclude a higher amount.

To charge or not to charge will soon be a moot question, if it is not already. With the current economic situation and the increasing knowledge of sound management and business practices, the days of anything gratis are short-lived. There is merit in charging even a token fee unless it is prohibited by the funding agent or continuing education is part of employee benefits, since people seem to value more an experience they have paid for. Considerations in pricing are past history of the program, competition, image, program objectives, audience, and finally, total program costs to determine the break-even point.

The philosophical dimension ought also be considered. Sometimes, although it is foreseen that any offering may not break even or make a profit, a decision is made to proceed with it; for instance, when pre-enrollment is unexpectedly low and it seems wiser to proceed and recover some of the money spent on planning; or when a future-oriented course not identified as a need by the nurse is offered; or when an expensive course with a clinical component is held for a few people because the market is small and/or it is believed that effective learning occurs best in a small class. If such a decision is made, the deficit must be made up from somewhere. One way is to schedule a mix of programs throughout the year that include several large profit-making conferences or "extravaganzas."

Effective pricing is probably the area of the mix in which continuing education administrators and providers are least comfortable, but more attention is being paid to it. Differential fees are given to members of professional associations and not to nonmembers. A few free places are allotted when an agency guarantees that a number of persons will attend. Certain types of offerings are priced differently per unit. It is worthwhile to consider how to price offerings and how to use pricing creatively in different ways to attract participants.

The Right Promotion

The right promotion means getting the essential information to the right people at the appropriate time. The objectives are to inform, to catch interest, and to be perceived as worthwhile to attend or purchase.

Promotion is not omnipotent. Other things can influence demand more than promotional activities, but promotion can inform the nurse of what is available and single out your organization and service from the maze of brochures now flooding the mail. The right kind of promotion will motivate that person to inquire or enroll.

Figure 10-1 lists components to consider when developing a brochure.

Figure 10.1 Brochure Components

Basic considerations
- Image
- Audience
- Program

Physical concerns
- Size—Economy of Printing and Mailing
- Color—Cost
  Judicious Use
- Design—Esthetic Appeal

Brochure cover
- Focus on Key Items
  - Title—Prominent Placement
  - Accreditation or Approval
  - Contact Hours
  - Date or Dates
  - Intended Audience
  - Length of Offering
  - Location

- Sponsor
- Tag Line—Why Attend?

Copy components
- What Will the Person Receive?
- What are the Benefits?
  Use support statements to explain, document
- How Does a Person Enroll?
- Any Cancellation Penalty?
- Any Payment Devices?
  - Bank Cards
  - Checks
  - Money Orders
- Any incentives?
  - Price Reduction
  - Special Events or Other Features

Mailing address section
- Urge to Share Brochure with Others
- Key items

Internal promotion. Promotion is directed externally and internally. It is important to build relationships with the internal publics: the dean or director of nursing or executive director; the continuing education or staff development staff and faculty; other deans and administrators in the university; and supervisory personnel on the hospital units. Keep them informed of your activities. Circulate reports to appropriate persons. Crucial questions of place in the structure of the organization, funding, and transfer of classroom information to application in practice depend on their support and cooperation.

Public relations. Public relations is an integral part of promotion. Top administrators spend a large part of their time attending meetings and receptions, participating in professional and public-service activities, serving on key committees, and seeking out funding sources. These situations all provide an opportunity to talk about the organization, to present the desired image, and to make contacts important to the future functioning of the unit. It is not just a cliche that the important business occurs during coffee breaks.

Methods. Promotional methods include the use of direct-mail brochures, fliers, or catalogs; calendar sections in publications; the direct approach through advisory boards or personal contact; news releases and advertising.

Each has certain advantages. Advertising is used to generate inquiries. Catalogs are best for broad, general listings of programs to a general or not easily identified audience, or one that is familiar with your organization, such as previous participants. Single brochures are best for promoting conferences, new or focused programs, or major events; they are also effective for reaching specific audiences for which mailing lists are available. Advisory boards are especially useful for specialty programs.

An effective mix, depending on the size and nature of the market, number and types of offerings, and money available might consist of a catalog for over fifteen courses, single brochures to reemphasize new programs and large conferences, and brief advertisements or news releases in the local nurses' association publication or the newspaper.

General promotional considerations are similar in different settings, but the scope and logistics of the task vary. Reaching the right person is literally the greatest challenge. Information may be stalled on someone's desk or discarded before the nurse sees it. Fliers are disregarded among numerous other brochures. Sometimes information is sent to persons unlikely to attend because insufficient thought was given to targeting the proper subgroup for mailing. Solving this problem is a greater challenge for a private provider or for a university-based continuing education department with a population of 20,000 than it would be for a small staff development unit that provides only for nurses in that agency or for a professional organization with a small, known membership. It becomes more complicated for staff development when programs are open to nurses in the community.

Cost. A balanced approach of neither under- or overpromoting is desired. In general, an average return of 2-3 percent enrollees can be expected from direct-mail promotion. Depending on the nature of the program and the nurse population, at some point the market might be saturated. Spending more on promotion would not provide more enrollees. By careful monitoring of money spent, methods used, and number and demographic characteristics of attendees, a provider can begin to promote efficiently.

The cost of marketing cannot be accurately assessed at this time. Marketing activities are defined differently in organization, and procedures for systematically tracking costs are sometimes limited. However, here are estimates of what some providers are spending: about 2.5 percent of departmental budget in a university-based continuing education in nursing unit; less than 1 percent of departmental budget for a hospital-based staff development unit or in-house continuing education type offerings; and 10 percent of gross for an independent provider. The percentage seems to be much higher for providers just beginning. How does this compare with what you are spending? Each unit needs to develop procedures, or use those of the host institution, to account for spending and to evaluate return on that investment.

Ethical issues. "Promoting your operation doesn't mean selling something you haven't got. It means building relationships. But relationships have to be built on substance [Lauffer 1977, p. 155]." Most organizations promote in a responsible way. They try to develop programs based on professional standards for continuing education programs, to advertise truthfully, to specify the benefits a participant can expect from the program, and, in general, to act as if they value their customers.

As education becomes more a lifelong learning process, providers of continuing education need to take a long-term view of their practices toward clients. Relationships are built over time. It takes a good deal of attention and care to build trust and to be seen as both responsive and responsible.

A few providers are not so scrupulous. Others are well intentioned but lack experience and qualifications. Nurses have complained about programs that were inferior, did not pertain to nursing, or were untruthfully advertised as approved or accredited.

Misleading advertising has other implications. There are misconceptions among legislators, the general public, and the nursing profession about the expectation that continuing education alone can guarantee competency. Providers must be especially careful not to promise results that are not feasible and, thereby, to reinforce the misconceptions.

Last, the cost of promotion is also an ethical consideration. Excessive or inefficient promotion usually means that the extra cost will be passed on to the consumer and/or the patient. It becomes doubly important to look at cost versus results and to assess the most effective promotion mix.

Consumer assistance. The number of providers of continuing education has burgeoned in the past five years, particularly in states that have mandatory continuing education. In California, more than 2800 providers had been approved by mid-1980 (California Board of Registered Nurses, personal communication). It is difficult for nurses to make choices among all these programs.

Articles and workshops have been developed to help the nurse be a more discriminating consumer. In her article, "Let the Buyer Beware," Curran (1978) suggests that nurses find out ahead of time about the provider, the faculty, program objectives and content, teaching methods, and approval by the board of registered nursing or the state nurses' association. Cooper (1979) suggests an excellent fourteen-question "Program Announcement Checklist" to evaluate the information about a program from a flier or brochure. Nurses still have a responsiblity to assess their needs, and to make any complaints afterward to the provider and/or to approval bodies.

From a slightly different perspective, O'Neal (1978) suggests ways for nursing administrators to maximize the return on their investment when they send an employee to continuing education offerings outside the hospital. She lists criteria to evaluate the quality of the offerings, suggests ways to ensure responsiveness to individual needs such as representation on advisory committees and adequate notices regarding conferences, and discusses criteria to determine staff participation in continuing education.

The Right Partners

Consumers and others such as employers, providers, and advisory committees can be very helpful in planning, promoting, and implementing programs. If chosen wisely, these sources offer valuable advice on program development, right location, and acceptable price. In turn, they may feel greater commitment to attending the program or assisting with its successful implementation. Members of advisory committees are often engaged to pave the way in the local area for an offering by building demand and acceptance (Lauffer 1977, pp. 159-160).

Evaluation

The marketing perspective continues through all program phases. Marketing information about program satisfaction and environment, unmet needs, suggestions for new programs, pertinent demographic information about participants, and how individuals heard about the program can be obtained from pre-, post-, and follow-up evaluation materials.

Marketing's Future Role

The rise of educational consumerism and the need for continuing education to be largely self-supporting will accentuate the need for quality marketing in the future (Frandson 1977). Other influencing factors will be competition, technology, information needs, and competency concerns.

Educational Consumerism

Rising consumerism in other parts of our lives is reflected in attitudes toward education. We have become a nation of adult learners, some of whom are quite vocal about their expectation and needs. To survive, organizations that choose to deliver educational services must be as responsibe as feasible and deliver quality services. If not, competitive providers will take over the market.

Self-support

Inflation, tax and budget cuts, the push for cost containment, and declining federal support indicate that continuing education will be mostly self-supporting in the future. Money for education competes with rapidly rising health and welfare costs, and the amount allotted for education is reduced accordingly. Therefore, continuing education cannot expect to see a reversal of current practices of little, if any, money appropriated at the state, local, and institutional levels.

Competition

Internal competition. Fiscal stringency will intensify competition for resources. Some nurses' associations are examining the actual cost of trying to provide continuing education for even a few members at a low price in relation to the amount of money available to achieve the rest of the organization's goals. These continuing education offerings will also need to be largely cost-effective.

As continuing education becomes more a part of the formal

organization in educational institutions, the expectation is that at least certain salaries will be paid. However, along with the status of a more formal position goes a loss of some of the autonomy that continuing education previously enjoyed, and more accountability to produce results and to justify money allocated.

External competition. Although mandatory continuing education has not gained great momentum, and a resurgence of students to fill educational institutions is expected after the turn of the century, continuing education will still be a necessary and potentially lucrative field. More and more providers, especially independent providers, are entering this field. Large numbers of providers split the market potential and the potential earnings for each provider. The result is pressure to find and keep clients, to diversify, and/or to form cooperative efforts.

Some providers have branched out into different products, such as independent study modules and publications. Others are merging efforts and sharing resources and planning decisions. However, large-scale, voluntary, cooperative efforts have not been particularly successful. Territoriality and private interests inhibit cooperative efforts. Other environmental factors or regulations may impose conditions that force more sharing. In the face of fiscal conservatism and competition, providers with marketing knowledge will have the edge.

Technology

Home videocassettes, satellites, computers with terminals for assisted instruction, and course-information systems all afford continuing education exciting ways to deliver services, advertise, and collect and distribute badly needed data about the field and its markets. Providers can cooperate with and use the knowledge and skills of firms that have large budgets for marketing. Sometimes, providers will have to compete with these firms and employ their own experts.

Information for Decisions

The organization. Providers need information from many sources to serve the community adequately. Each organization needs to develop communication systems to feed information in from the outside about nurses and trends, and to deliver information externally to consumers and other pertinent groups. It does not need to be elaborate, but it must be systematic.

The consumer. Most of us suffer from information overload. As providers and courses keep proliferating, and rapid social and technological changes occur, ways must be sought to organize and disseminate information most effectively. Regional, computerized information systems, such as the model developed by the Western Regional Center for Continuing Education in Nursing at the University of California in San Francisco, are one alternative. These systems can perform many functions, such as gathering information about courses and producing catalogs for nurses, analyzing data from needs assessments, and compiling demographic and management information for providers and policymakers. For smaller areas, calendars work well if providers submit listings. Nurses would very much like to have a central place to get information instead of making many phone calls or, in some cases, remaining uninformed.

Competency Concerns

The continuing concern about practitioner competency is focusing more concretely on performance measures and ways to assess practice-related needs. In addition to observation, the availability of streamlined ways for nurses to assess their own needs and for counseling and referral services to match needs to programs will become more necessary. Computerized self-assessment inventories and a program-referral system have been developed by the University of Texas Health Science Center School of Nursing at San Antonio's Multi-Faceted Program for Continuing Education in Nursing (1977). Other methods might include personal consultation for a fee or as part of a department's services.

Conclusion

Marketing is an orientation and an approach to the stages of programming. Although they may not be aware of it, providers of continuing education in nursing do perform marketing functions. These functions will need to be more formal and systematic in the future when environmental conditions such as consumerism, competition, and financial concerns demand that organizations be able to research needs skillfully, promote effectively, efficiently, and honestly, and deliver high-quality programs.

Larger units may develop a marketing staff or use expertise and facilities provided through the host institution. Other providers may rely on their past experience, attend workshops, or learn from consultants and do their own marketing. Still others may simply contract out their marketing work. Whatever methods are employed, each administrator, coordinator, and independent provider must understand the concepts of marketing and how to use them to the advantage of their organization and their consumers.

References

Benner, Richard V. "How to Get a Good Thing Going: Marketing Continuing Education in Nursing." Presented at the Annual Conference on Continuing Education in Nursing, Boston, October 31-November 1, 1977, pp. 1-3.

Buchanan, W. Wray, and Barksdale, H.C. "Marketing's Broadening Concept is Real in University Extension." *Adult Education* 25(1): 34-35, 1974.

Calderon, Jewell R. "Marketing Your Program." *Journal of Continuing Education in Nursing* 9(3):13, May-June 1978.

Cooper, Signe S. "How to Make the Proper CE Selection: Think Before You Buy!" *CE Focus* 2(1):4-5, January-February 1979.

Curran, Connie. "Factors Affecting Participation in CE Activities and Identified Learning Needs of Registered Nurses." *Journal of Continuing Education in Nursing* 8(4):18-22, July-August 1977.

Curran, Connie. "Let the Buyer Beware." *Journal of Continuing Education in Nursing* 9(5):11-13, September-October, 1978.

Del Bueno, Dorothy J. "Viewpoint: CE: Treatment for Outdatedness." *Nursing Administration Quarterly* 2(2):63, Winter 1978.

Frandson, Phillip E. "Basic Building Blocks for Century's End Continuing Education." *Adult Leadership* 25(10):291, 321, June 1977.

Kotler, Philip. *Marketing for Nonprofit Organizations.* Englewood Cliffs, N.J.: Prentice-Hall, 1975. p. 5.

Lauffer, Armand. *The Practice of Continuing Education in the Human Services.* New York: McGraw-Hill, 1977, pp. 151-162.

Multi-Faceted Program for Continuing Education in Nursing: Final Progress Report. The University of Texas Health Science Center at San Antonio School of Nursing, September 1977.

O'Neal, Ellen A. "Maximize the Return on Your Investment." *Journal of Continuing Education in Nursing* 9(4):21-23, July-August 1978.

Thompson, James D. *Organizations in Action.* New York: McGraw-Hill, 1967, p. 13.

Bibliography

Cooper, Signe S., et al. "Nursing Administration Quarterly Forum: Continuing Education." *Nursing Administration Quarterly* 2(2): 73-81, Winter 1978.

Kuramoto, Alice M. "Mind over Matter: How to Make an Intelligent CE Choice." *CE Focus* 2(1):6-7, January-February 1979.

Murphy, Marion I. "The Continuing Education Program from the Perspective of a Dean." *Journal of Continuing Education in Nursing* 9(3):48-51, May-June 1978.

Vavrek, Michael. "Marketing: It's OK—We're OK." *Adult Leadership* 25(4):101-102, 118, December 1976.

This chapter is reprinted from *Perspectives on Continuing Education in Nursing*, edited by Signe S. Cooper, RN, FAAN, and Margo C. Neal, RN, MN. Nurseco, Inc.: Pacific Palisades, CA.

11

Networking: Plugging Into the Right Connections

Mary-Scott Welch

As you consider going into business, there is a single technique that you can apply that can make all the difference. This technique, which is easy to learn and fun to use, can open doors you may never have thought to knock on, and it can give you the kind of down-to-earth, specific information you'll need.

The word for this technique is one you may already have heard bandied about, for it reflects what Betty Friedan has called "one of the best new developments of the women's movement." The word is *networking,* and it is something that can enrich and inform your entire career.

Networking in Action

The way I discovered the networking phenomenon is an example of how networking really works. *Redbook* magazine had asked me to write an article to be called "The Ten Best Corporations for Women to Work For." I assumed that every corporation on the Fortune 500 list would be beating on my door, wanting to make *Redbook's* ten best list, so before starting my research I worked out a list of criteria they'd have to meet.

First of all, they'd have to have a good, strong affirmative action program—meaning they were going out of their way to recruit, hire, train, and promote women as never before.

Second they'd have to show me figures to prove that their affirmative action plan was really working—for example, that they now had more women in management than before, and more women on career ladders that could lead to management.

Well, a funny thing happened when I went out to do my interviews for this article: The public relations people were nice as pie to me—that's their job—but they skirted around my questions in a mysterious way. Instead of giving me the numbers I needed, they wanted me to interview their stars—you know, the first woman this and the first woman that. (We were all tired of that kind of story by that time; this was 1976 or 1977.) Or they wanted to give me percentages: "We have 100 percent more women in management this year than last," they'd say. Well, you know what that could mean. It could mean two women managers instead of one.

I was getting desperate about this assignment when a wonderful thing happened: I met a woman who worked in one of these corporations I was trying to find out about, and she did *not* work in public relations. Call her Jane. "*My* company doesn't belong on any ten best list," she said, "but I hear they're doing pretty well over at X Company. Call my friend Cindy over there. She'll tell you what's going on." I called Cindy and she said, "I can't talk now. Here's my home phone." So I called her at home, and then she not only gave me the inside story about her corporation but said, "Call Alice over at Y Company. Tell her I said to call." Alice passed me on to Ruth, who referred me to Mary and—you see what was happening? I was being plugged into a nationwide, informal network of working women who were talking to each other behind the scenes. They were talking to each other across company lines, across occupational lines, and across the hierarchical lines that so often seem to keep us apart in the workaday world—and these women were talking to *me*, whom they didn't even know, giving me information and insights I couldn't get any other way, simply because Cindy told me to call Alice who told me to call Ruth—and so on. And it all began because I happened to meet Jane. That's networking.

In my case these women were helping me get my job done, but they might just as well have been helping me to *find* a job, to set up a new business, or to put me in contact with key people who would buy my products or services. They might have been giving me moral support in some battle I was waging. Or they might have been getting their power together to affect corporation or government policy. All those possibilities are inherent in the simplest of networking connections.

And that's what I wrote about, in the end. I didn't write "The Ten Best Corporations"—there weren't any. I wrote, "How Women Just Like You Are Getting Together to Get Better Jobs." (Interestingly enough, I used the word *network* only once in that whole article, but that's what it was all about: women networking, women helping each other in the work world.)

The Process of Networking

Networking is the process of developing business contacts that you can use for information, advice, referrals, and moral support as you expand your career. Women's networking, a nationwide phenomenon, is our answer to the informal but influential system that customarily leaves women out, the "old boys' " network. In old boys' networks, men throw business, job leads, and crucial inside information to former classmates or teammates, golf partners, and other males whom they know better or feel more comfortable with than with us relative newcomers to the business and professional ranks.

To understand networking, it helps to form a mental picture of the technique. Picture yourself in the center of a huge, farflung fisherman's net. Imagine that each knot in the net is a person. You are directly connected with only those knots or people immediately surrounding you, such as your parents and other relatives, your peers, your colleagues, physicians, babysitters, neighbors, and acquaintances in your home community. None of those are business contacts in the strict sense of the term, but all of them have and can introduce you to business contacts of their own. Through skillful networking, I firmly believe you could be introduced to the President of the United States.

But you needn't reach that far in the net. The people you want to talk to are people who have had direct experience with business, people who can refer you to potential advisers; nurses who are already in business.

Start the networking process by asking the knots nearest you if they know any sources that have the information you need. And don't decide in advance that the answer will be no. For all you know, your homemaker mother's former roommate may now be president of an insurance agency and possessor of an address book laden with phone numbers that you can call in her name. The husband of one of your colleagues may be just the person who can give you a plethora of resources and information that will help you. These people can help you only if you let them know what contacts you are looking for and why.

Since I first discussed the phenomenon, networking has become a lot more organized, but it's still a matter of women *talking* to each other, or women banding together for mutual support.

Here's how the process might begin: You and I meet at a nursing seminar. You know 100 people, and I know 100 people. They don't know each other. They just know you . . . and me . . . but now we've met, you and I, so now we can connect your 100 with my 100. Just because they know you, and me, now they can know each other.

But that's only the beginning, because each of your 100 knows another 100, who know another 100, and so on. Picture that network of interconnections! Its possibilities are practically limitless!

In our case, still at the nursing seminar, what might happen next? Well, suppose you were thinking of going into midwifery, and you wanted to talk to someone about whether it was better to work through a hospital or go into joint practice—or what? You might ask me and say, "Do you know anyone who's in joint practice as a midwife?"

Actually, I'm not the sort of person you want in your network. You want to know other nurses, other health professionals, politicians, administrators, and so on, but in networking you never know who knows what until you ask. And, as it happens, I *could* put you in touch with a filmmaker who just completed a documentary on midwifery, and so probably knows everyone in the field. If you called *her*, using my name, she'd knock herself out to help you. That's networking.

Or, suppose I called you and said, "I'm doing an article on nurse/doctor relations. Do you know anyone who has some war stories to tell, in confidence, of course?" If you didn't know the perfect interviewee for me, you'd probably know someone who did. You'd plug me into your network of nurses, and doctors. I'd call and say *you* referred me. That's networking.

But . . . we wouldn't do that for each other (I wouldn't give you the filmmaker's number, and you wouldn't plug me into my network) if we'd only just met. So a big part of networking is getting to *know* other women—getting to know their capabilities, their interests, their background; getting to know how they fit into your plans and how you can fit into theirs; developing trust and confidence in each other.

And this doesn't happen overnight.

How *does* it happen?

Well, first you meet another woman—at a nursing convention, in a continuing education program, even in the cafeteria or the supermarket. You introduce yourselves. You exchange business cards. You tell each other about your work, slipping in your credentials. (Don't be afraid to brag a little.) Maybe you discuss a problem that's common to all nurses—the image problem or working conditions, or pay, perhaps.

Next you follow up on that meeting. You call the new person and make a date to talk further, or you send a clipping on the subject discussed. Maybe you invite her to a meeting that will interest her. The object is to get to know her better, so you'll know *whom* she knows and *what* she knows, next time you need someone to call for information, for advice, for a referral—or whatever.

Eventually, she becomes an important part of your network, and you are an important part of hers. You know just how to use each other, for your mutual benefit.

Now don't balk at that word *use*. The members of your network are going to use you just as much as you use them. You are a *resource* for others, and the sooner you realize that, the more comfortable you'll be with this whole process. You'll start offering your help—freely, generously—knowing that it will come back to you in one way or another. It always does. Men have proven this; they have been networking successfully for years.

This concept of networking is new to a lot of women. It's a whole new feeling, a whole new attitude. Many of us were trained to *compete* with each other, rather than *help* each other. In the first place we were competing for men—but this isn't about men; it's about work.

Well, sometimes it *is* about men, and how we behave around men—unconsciously, for the most part. Sometimes we have to learn to support other women, consciously, in spite of our conditioning.

Edith Seashore, a top-notch management consultant whose accomplishments include integrating women into the US Naval Academy, told me a story that illustrates that point. She was then the president of the National Training Labs, and one of only two women on a particular board of directors. The other woman on the board had opinions, an agenda, and even a personality at opposite poles from Edith's own; they couldn't have been less alike. But after a few meetings Edith noticed that every time the other woman spoke up, the men only pretended to listen. As soon as she stopped talking, the men seemed to go on with their own meeting as though she'd never opened her mouth. So even though she herself tended not to agree with what Ms. Jones was apt to suggest to the meeting, Edith began saying things like, "I think the board might like to hear more about what you have in mind, Ms. Jones," or "Are you satisfied with the board's response to your comment?" or even, to the men, "Just a minute: I'm not sure Ms. Jones has finished what she wants to say." Soon—without their even having discussed this between themselves—the other woman was doing the same for Edith. They were deliberately supporting each other. In effect, they were supporting the right of women to *be* there. But, as Edith told me, "I had to *learn* to do that. I had to make myself do it. It just wasn't natural, at first."

Natural or not, women supporting other women is the essence of networking. And when they see how it works, how cooperating achieves so much more than *competing* ever did, women build networking into every aspect of their lives.

Let me give you some examples of how this system has worked for women I interviewed. These examples are from the business world, and the situations may seem very different from the type you encounter in nursing, but look for the technique, the process, the spirit of networking, in these stories. Those aspects don't change, from office to academia to hospital.

Take the case of Kate Rand Lloyd, for instance. Her story could apply to you if you ever decided to change jobs, or move out of nursing altogether, and the only people you knew were the ones you worked with in your present position.

Kate Lloyd is now the editor-in-chief of *Working Woman* magazine. She was at *Vogue*, as articles editor, when she realized she was stuck (yes, women can get stuck at upper levels, and in glamorous fields, too). At the same time, she realized that she knew hardly a soul outside Conde Nast, the firm that publishes *Vogue, Glamour,* and so on. "It was like a convent there," Kate told me. She knew she had to start getting out and around. She had to make herself visible.

She did it through a very deliberate plan of networking, beginning with two women who had also started out with Vogue, many years before, but were now involved in politics and in volunteer work. They introduced her into their separate circles, to the point where one day Betty Harris, then the publisher of *Working Woman*, said to volunteer Kate (who was frantically putting out a daily paper for delegates to the Democratic National Convention), "When this is all over, let's have lunch." (In New York, at least, those are key words in networking: "Let's have lunch.") The rest is history— and I don't mean Democratic history—but from her top of the heap at *Working Woman*, Kate points out this crucial fact: "It took me two years." Moral: Start networking *before* you feel any specific need to. Start building a network outside the place where you work so it will be ready when (if) you need it. Start now to make yourself visible in your profession, beyond your immediate job. (One way to do both is to become active in your professional organizations.)

Or consider the story Lore Caulfield told me. This could apply to you if you have an idea you think you might develop into a business—a new product, a service, maybe some improvement in health care delivery.

Lore Caulfield is now the head of a million-dollar business. Do you know Lore Lingerie? Precious stuff, very precious, sold at such fancy stores as Neiman Marcus and Bergdorf Goodman. But at the time she experienced the wonders of networking she was a full-time television producer with NBC in Los Angeles; making beautiful underwear was a little sideline for her, a "cottage industry" as she put it. Then a $5000 shipment of silk was due in, and she didn't have the money to pay for it. (I believe this is called a cash-flow problem.) Just complaining to her network, never expecting anything more than sympathy, Lore was knocked flat when they passed the hat—for a 90-day loan that no bank would have touched.

"It wasn't so much the money," she told me, "although that was absolutely crucial at the time. It was the trust their confidence in me."

But I think my favourite example, of all the hundreds I keep in my collection, is that of Constance Cook. Constance Cook got the inside information from her network, a network she didn't even know she had.

She was about to interview for the job of vice-president for land-grant affairs at Cornell University, but she had no idea what salary to ask for. . . when in the mail, anonymously, she received a printout on salary ranges for the job. She got the job, and when she arrived at her desk, on her first day, she found a vase of roses with the card, "Congratulations, from your network."

It turns out they were the secretaries in the office. They wanted a woman in that job, and particularly *this* woman—a former state legislator known as a battler for women's rights.

Types of Networks

As I mentioned, networking has become a lot more organized than it was when I lucked onto the movement. All over the country, women have been organizing groups for the sole purpose of networking. These groups are in addition to the old-line professional organizations.

They come in all sizes—a little group of ten, which is actually more of a support group, and one that's so big it might warrant that remark of Yogi Berra's about a restaurant. He said, "Nobody goes there any more. It's too crowded."

Network names range from the definitive—Women In Government Relations, for instance—to the mysterious: MAD. (It stands for Men Are Dumb.)

These networks are *internal* or *external*—that is, they're organized inside the place where the women work, or they meet outside, cutting across institutional lines. Both types have their advantages and disadvantages. I'd belong to both, if I were you—in fact, I'd belong to as many different kinds as I could locate—but the naive should be cautioned; a good networker operates differently in different kinds of networks.

Whether internal or external, networks may also be *vertical* or *horizontal*—that is, in a vertical network, anyone at any level of the career ladder is welcome to join; a horizontal network is more of a peer group, limiting its membership to women who work at about the same level: they're all supervisors or educators, say, or all clinical specialists.

Both vertical and horizontal networks have their points. Kati Sasseville, one of the founders of AGOG, in Minneapolis, put the case for the vertical network, which AGOG definitely is. (AGOG stands for All the Good Old Girls, and I do believe that all the good old girls in St. Paul and Minneapolis must belong to it!) "In an exclusive group," Kati said, "one day you need to hire someone at the entry level, and your network doesn't reach down that far. But our network also reaches up, so it can help if your problem is, say, the governor just cut your budget $20,000 for a very important project, and you need to talk to him.''

As for the horizontal network, well, it saves time when one inservice person can talk to another inservice person, someone who's having the same kind of problems, without having to explain all the background, as might be necessary if a clinical person were sitting in. Besides, women who are cast as "role models" sometimes get tired of the role. As one executive women said to me, smiling but obviously weary, "I gave at the office."

Sometimes the horizontal network is accused of being elitist, and that's a bad word among feminists. But there's another way to look at the practice of *selecting* members. The president of a San Francisco network put it this way: "We're open to every woman who has made it!"

Whether vertical or horizontal, some networks limit themselves to a particular occupation: for example, women in communications. In New York, the Financial Women's Association is important; there is a national network of affirmative action officers.

Then there are the underground networks; most, as you might imagine, are in-house networks. They don't want their managements to know they exist. (Some managements are indeed suspicious when women get together. They're afraid of unionization, or of sex discrimination suits, as well they might be: some of the greatest breakthroughs that women have made in corporations have come about through the women's networks that brought suits—and won!)

In certain corporations, though, networks have their management's blessing. Take the networks at Equitable Life, for example. In contrast to the network at NBC, where the women weren't even allowed to use the bulletin boards—they posted notices of their meetings on the mirrors in the ladies room, and even then, half the time found they'd been torn down—networks at Equitable have use of corporate facilities, from meeting rooms to copy machines, *and* an official budget.

Beginnings

For all the variety of the networks I've met, most of them began in exactly the same way: one woman had the idea . . . she talked to another woman about the need . . . next time they met, each brought in another woman . . . and soon they had a steering committee for a complete network. To cite a few examples:

- Nancy Korman started the Women's Lunch Group, in Boston, because she was mad. She had done a lot of political favors for a man in the construction business, but when she called him with an eye to soliciting his account for her graphics firm, he turned her down flat."Oh," he said, "I give all my printing business to a man who belongs to my men's club."

  Nancy thought, "While I'm doling out snap, crackle, and pop, he's making business deals." She told three other women she knew what had happened, and the Lunch Group was under way. (I guess it's a lunch group, rather than a breakfast club, because the women still have to dole snap, crackle, and pop— but no matter: they're organized to do business with each other.)

- Diane Winokur started the Bay Area Executive Women's Forum, in San Francisco, because she had the hunch that women managers were way ahead of the books and articles being printed about them. She wrote to ten or fifteen management women to see if they felt the same. They did, as they agreed over lunch. A year and a half later, their network had 100 dues-paying members.

- Sudy Blumenthal (now Forman) started the River Oaks Breakfast Club, in Houston, because she was new in town, didn't know any other women, and was, in her word, "terrified." Typically, the club had more applicants than it could accommodate—so spin-off groups started up.

Multiply these examples by hundreds—maybe thousands—and you see why Betty Friedan said, "Networking gives every woman new strength and support and shows her how to make equal opportunity work for her despite the old boys' network" (Welch 1980).

Speaking of the old boys' network, you may be amused to know that when I first began talking about it, and how it leaves women out, the "old boy" I live with (my husband) told me there was no such thing. He wasn't putting me on. A lot of men still say that. I think it's because they've been doing what they do for so long, and doing it so naturally, that they don't have to give it a name. (But oh, how they do it! And oh, how it works!)

Rules of the System

There are a few dos and don'ts that will make your networking more successful—and help the system keep growing, for all of us:

1. Do put in as much as you take out of this system. Networking is not a gimme-gimme system. It's more of a you-scratch-my-back-I'll-scratch-yours system, and it works best is you do *your* scratching first. That is, offer your help before you ask for help for yourself. Be generous.

2. Do be meticulous about getting back to anyone who gives you a lead. Report on what happened. Do this immediately after a phone call or interview or whatever, but remember to do it later, too, when the deal finally goes through or you have further contact with the source your networker has given you. (Sometimes this may be *years* later, so it pays to keep good records of your networking.) Or, if someone referred a client to you, do send a short note to thank her for the referral and to affirm that the client did come to see you.

3. Do listen to advice when you've asked for it. Don't say, even if true, "I though of that," or "I tried that, and it didn't work." You don't have to *do* what your adviser suggests, but at least listen, and consider; don't stomp on ideas.

4. Don't expect too much, too soon, from your network. Networking is magic, but it's not *instant* magic. Network for the long haul, for the *future* that you and the women and the other nurses you meet are going to live out. I recently had the happy experience of seeing two women take that advice, right on the spot. I had addressed a new network in Vancouver, British Columbia. Afterwards, the sponsors had an autograph party for my book. I was busily signing books when one young woman—she couldn't have been more than twenty-five—asked me to write, in hers, "To the first woman Prime Minister of Canada." While I was saying "I hope you make it," another young woman stepped out of the line, held up her business card, and cried out, "She'll make it! I'll manage her campaign."

5. Lastly, do take the initiative in your networking. Don't sit on your hands and wait for someone to come up to you at a meeting. Go introduce yourself, circulate, then follow up, and keep in touch.

You know, they say there are three kinds of people: Those who make things happen, those who watch what's happening, and those who can only say, "What happened?"

Networking makes things happen. But *you have to make networking happen.*

Here's to your success in doing just that!

Reference

Welch, Mary-Scott. *Networking: The Great New Way for Women to Get Ahead*. New York: Harcourt Brace Jovanovich, 1980 ($9.95); New York: Warner Books, 1981 ($2.95).

12

Going with the Risk

Joan Reighley

And when he came to the place where the wild things are they roared their terrible roars and gnashed their terrible teeth and rolled their terrible eyes and showed their terrible claws till Max said "BE STILL" and tamed them with the magic trick of staring into their yellow eyes without blinking once. —Maurice Sendak, 1963.

Each of us has our "wild things"—situations, behaviors, and places that seem scary and full of risk. There is a fine edge of excitement, exhilaration, and creative learning when we dare to go with the risk and explore these wild things. Going with the risk leads to the growing edge, the crisis place of danger and opportunity. Risk is inherent in any new venture. Entering the world of business is an adventure and a transition or crisis where danger and opportunity abound.

I would like to share with you my experience and ideas about the process of risking, including choice and responsibility, change, how we stop ourselves, holding on and letting go, alternatives to scaring yourself, and getting in touch with personal power. I will discuss risk, change, and strategies for risking as applied to going into business.

The Process of Risking

Choice and Responsibility

Human beings have the ability to solve problems, make choices, and act with intent. In this way we are responsible for ourselves and our personal environment. Responsibility equals the *ability* to respond. To choose with responsibility and self-awareness, we must be centered and able to focus on our own feelings, hopes, ideals, attitudes, and reservations. "Human freedom involves our capacity to pause between stimulus and response, and, in that pause, to choose the one response toward which we wish to throw our weight. The capacity to create ourselves, based on this freedom, is inseparable from consciousness or self-awareness" (May 1975).

Self-creation is an awesome responsibility and a challenge. It may be helpful to remember that with the freedom to make choices and take the consequences, we also have the freedom to change our choice, to make mistakes and learn from them, and to start again. Self-creation can be thought of in terms of a dynamic trial run; in a trial run, there is no such thing as a right or wrong way, or a mistake. There is an expectation of many alternative ways, with differing consequences; some alternatives will work better than others, and almost all will have to be modified depending on the unique situation. The trial run concept avoids the paralyzing dichotomies of good or bad, right or wrong, black or white; risk is minimized in the dynamic process of choosing and creating.

The limitations of human freedom include the individual's response to change, expectations of self and own abilities, and variables of culture, religion, socialization, and consideration of significant others. These limitations include "shoulds" and "don'ts" as well as "I can't"; risking a creative look at the self-imposed limitations to freedom can lead to responsible growth and change.

How We Stop Ourselves
We human beings stop ourselves from choosing, from risking, and we limit our freedom of choice in an infinite variety of ways. Take a moment to be aware of your reservations about going into business for yourself. To increase your awareness, complete these sentences on a piece of paper or in your mind:

- Nurses are supposed to—
- Nurses should—
- Nurses shouldn't—
- Nurses can't—
- Women are supposed to—
- Women should—

- Women shouldn't—
- Women can't—
- I'm supposed to—
- I should—
- I shouldn't—
- I can't—

Compare your list with this list:

- Nurses are supposed to take care of sick people, serve the doctor, wear white and work in a hospital, work long hours and not complain, always be clean and competent.
- Nurses shouldn't bring their feelings to work, complain, get rich, be in business for themselves, strike.
- Nurses can't have a private practice, work for themselves, be businesswomen, write their own ticket, make diagnoses.
- I don't know how; I can't learn. I'm not a leader. I'll go broke. I'm not enough; somebody else does it better. Someone else is already doing it. I'll be illegal, immoral, selfish. I'll be all alone. They'll find out I can't do it; I'm a fake. I'm ordinary. If I am successful, men will be threatened and reject me; women will be jealous and snub me. I can't win.

Doubts, negative thoughts and images, and "shoulds" are some of the ways we stop ourselves from risking new ways of being; each of us has a litany of old tapes that replay themselves when we are threatened by risking a new behavior or choice. Examples of "shoulds" include "Nurses should work for hospitals, clinics, or doctors," "Nurses should wear caps," "Nurses should wear white uniforms." We scare ourselves by going with the doubt, the negative thought or image, or the "should", usually because of habit and the lack of another response or belief, image, or should that is positive and up-to-date with our present reality. We stop ourselves by believing the old tape.

Holding On and Letting Go

Holding on to the past is a common way we stop ourselves. An example can be found in the Bible: Lot's wife disobeyed God's order not to look back; she turned her eyes and her thoughts toward her past, a decadent and crumbling city. The story states that God punished her by turning her into a pillar of salt. In holding on to the past, Lot's wife lost her chance to move into the future.

Living creatures must grow and change to live. There is no staying the same, or living in the past, for to stay the same is to begin to die. Our choice as humans is to live or die; there is no almost or sort of alive just as there is no almost or sort of pregnant. You either are or you aren't. Living is a dynamic process of unfolding and changing; to stay the same is to regress, to go backwards, to begin to die. Some people are walking around dead inside, staying the same, looking alive only from a distance, a facade of aliveness, like a mannequin in a store window that *almost* looks alive.

Picture the Dead Sea or the great Salt Lake; from a distance, both appear to be blue, alive bodies of water. Both are dead and do not support life. Why? They are dead or closed systems. Systems theory tells us that living, open systems continuously exchange energy with the environment. Dead, closed systems do not exchange energy and are stopped or plugged up; the dynamic life-giving flow of energy with the environment has stopped. Either no energy or input comes into the system, or no energy or output goes out of the system.

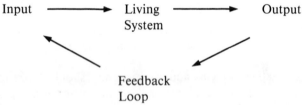

Figure 12-1

Each individual can be thought of as a living system, as can a family, an organization, a health care team, or any individual or collection of living beings. Take a moment to become aware of your life experience with closed systems. Think of a person you know who does not choose to change. How do you experience this person? Describe this person. What is exciting and interesting about her? Do you look forward to spending time with her? How much time do you spend with her? Why? How does this person see you? Does this person accept new ideas? Does this person have much fun?

Think of an organization that has remained the same for years; describe how the organization functions, what its management and communication patterns are, how effective it is. What are the organizational procedures and rules? Are they effective? How do you fit in with this organization? How do you feel about working for or with it? Can you be yourself, wear your usual clothes, be spontaneous? Do you find you have to play a role? How accepting of new ideas is the organization? In what ways do you observe this organization holding on to the past?

Individuals and organizations have many reasons for holding on to the past; most of them have a commonality of choosing safety and security—or the *illusion* of safety and security. We human beings tend to hold on to past ways of being because past ways are known ways; new ways of being are unknown. We hold on for dear life, literally.

We imagine the unknown as a dark jungle, an unknown planet; perhaps we will fall off the edge of the earth or get eaten by dragons. We imagine that we will not be able to cope in the unknown; "I don't like what I've got, but at least I can handle it." We tend to hold on to boring and stagnant old patterns rather than choose to let go of the known and go into the unknown.

New behaviors and patterns seem difficult and awkward, uncomfortable. To increase your awareness of the difficulty of new behaviors, write with your nondominant hand; eat dinner with chopsticks. Remember how it was for you to learn to ride a bicycle, use roller skates, type, give an injection, or carry out any nursing procedure.

Other reasons for holding on to the past may be that some of the past patterns worked well and were effective; also involved are respect for history and tradition, respect for authority figures, shaping, and early patterns that were set and accepted without evaluation in the here and now.

Letting go is risky; yet human beings know how to let go, just as human beings know how to hold on. Take a moment to remember scenes from childhood in which you took a risk and let go. I can remember:

- Wanting to be a big girl and ride my bike without training wheels
- Standing on a diving board, wanting to dive in head first
- Swinging from a rope across a pool of water like Tarzan
- Letting my kitten play outside by himself; hoping he would be safe and find his way back home
- Writing a poem in school and showing it to my teacher and the class, not knowing for sure whether they would like it or laugh
- Wanting to sing in the chorus, but not wanting to audition

Going from childhood to adolescence involves a great deal of risk. Let yourself focus on the transitions in your teenage years; what did you experience as you went from grade school to junior high? If you are willing, write down some of your experiences from adolescence. I remember leaving grade school, with the safety of one classroom, one teacher, one group of students, and my own desk that I did not have to share, and graduating into an unknown junior high with six different periods, classrooms, teachers, and classes of students; my hall locker and my gym locker had combination locks on them, and I could not remember the combinations—was it 34-12-22 left-right-left, or right-left-right?

Common risks from adolescence include:

- Daring to separate from family to form a peer group
- Letting go of same sex group socialization to include opposite sex friends
- Dating and having relationships with the opposite sex
- Daring to be different from the peer group and express unique self values and behaviors
- Learning to drive a car
- Working for the first time outside the family
- Leaving home, with the ambivalence of wanting support emotionally and financially while craving independence and freedom.

The risks and predictable growth and development of adult life have been well described by Gail Sheehy in *Passages: Predictable Crises of Adult Life,* and Edna LeShan in *The Wonderful Crisis of Middle Age.*

The courage to take new steps allows us to let go of each stage with its satisfactions and to find the fresh responses that will release the richness of the next. The power to animate all of life's seasons is a power that resides within us. [Sheehy 1976, p. 354]

Middle age can offer the greatest risks of all, but if you have the courage to take the necessary leap into faith, the adventure can be the most important and wonderful one that you can ever experience. [LeShan 1973, p. 13]

Each developmental stage has these places of choice: shall I hold on to the past, known situation, or shall I let go of the known and go into the unknown, the void, the vacuum? The unknown is anticipated as a void or vacuum; the void has been defined as "empty space, vacuum, opening, gap, containing nothing" (Webster, 1973). Therein lies the paradox of the unknown, for in modern physics, the vacuum is a space of infinite potential power. "The physical vacuum—as it is called in field theory—is not a state of mere nothingness, but contains the potentiality for all forms of the particle world . . . the discovery of the dynamic quality of the vacuum is seen by many physicists as one of the most important findings of modern physics" (Capra 1977, p. 209).

We can play with some paradoxical ideas:

No-thing is every-thing.
There is no donut without a hole.
Eat up the donut and you still have the hole.
There is no way to know the unknown, for when it is known, it
    is no longer unknown.
There is no way to prepare yourself for the unknown and yet all
    your life experience prepared you; at any moment, you
    are prepared and unprepared simultaneously.

Going into the void, the vacuum, the unknown, is an adventure with excitement and risk of the unexpected, for we cannot know what to expect in the unknown; potentially, anything can happen. And we cannot know about the unknown until we take the risk to go into the unknown, the leap of faith in ourselves and in life as a dynamic process. This leap of faith is a surrender to life process, a "yes"to the growing edge of our life force.

The nurse who decides to go into business for herself must risk letting go of known ways of being and supporting herself and take some steps into the unknown. I'd like to share with you some of my own experiences from when I was deciding to go into business for myself as a mental health counselor in private practice. My thoughts and feelings were a jumble of realistic concerns and questions, plus some old fears and new excitement:

- How can I let go of my full-time job and still pay my bills?
- Is my malpractice insurance adequate?
- What if I get sued?

- What about my health insurance, retirement?
- What happens if I get sick and can't work?
- What bookkeeping method shall I use?
- Shall I do my bookkeeping and filing myself
  or pay to have it done?
- How will I get third-party payment?
- Can I really make it in private practice?

I found myself holding on to old ways of being, clinging to old, known roles, and resisting new ways of being.

- I kept "forgetting" to order business cards: after all, I'd lived my whole life without them and didn't really need them.
- I continued to use informal stationery, without a letterhead.
- I had a difficult time discussing fees and a contract for paying fees.
- I invited a psychologist friend to share office space, and offered him the larger, lighter office.

I especially found myself holding on to the illusion that I was safer, financially and professionally, if I was working for an institution. The illusion included belief that the institution would take care of me with monthly paychecks, retirement, health insurance, sick leave, and job security in case of nationwide financial depression. There was also a sense of being a legitimate professional if I worked within an agency or institution. I was aware that to get this job security, I had to meet the institution's needs and mandates, which could change in a way that would conflict with my needs and values. I call this phenomenon bureaucratic or civil service mentality, and I find these illusions running rampant in nurses and in others who work for someone else, whether they work in a doctor's office or clinic, or in an institutional setting.

Remembering this process of holding on and letting go, I am amazed and respectful of the powerful process of risk taking and change; as I compare my own experiences to the experiences of others, I am struck by the commonalities and the universality of the risk-taking process. The ability to step into the unknown is developed by keeping in mind the positive aspects of risk and by learning strategies to deal with risk.

Positive Aspects of Risk Taking

Let yourself focus for a moment on the positive aspects of risk taking in your life experience. What were the feelings that you experienced in your childhood when you dared to go with the risk? The positive aspects might include any of the following:

- The joy of discovery
- Creativity
- Curiosity
- A sense of wonder
- Unexpected pleasure and fun
- Relief of boredom
- Adventure
- Surprise
- Accomplishment
- Being avante-garde, ahead of your time; the first one on the block to do something
- Being special, envied, different, one up
- Knowing what you want and going for it
- Getting what you want

And there is much, much more; the positive aspects to risk taking are infinite in number and unique to each individual. These positive aspects lead to change and growth; the positive aspects motivate and energize one to self-actualization and re-creation of spirit.

The Process of Change

Change is an ongoing process. People will change behaviors and attitudes to meet the basic needs of life: safety, belongingness, close love relationships, respect, prestige, food, clothing, and shelter. People will change to reduce anxiety; we human beings are fearful of the unknown, the unfamiliar, the unexpected. There is a motivation to change in crisis, to alleviate the discomfort of anxiety or intense feelings. People will change to meet developmental needs and potential for creativity or pleasure.

During change there is an accompanying sense of loss; as the individual or group changes, the stages of the loss process become manifest: shock and disbelief, denial, "not me"; the intense feelings that go with developing awareness of loss, anger, fear, guilt, sadness, depression, "why me?" Because of this, there is much resistance to change. If this resistance is ignored, it will persist and block or slow down the change process. To facilitate change, the resistance to change must be acknowledged by the individual who wants to change; the resistance represents very good reasons, unique to the individual, to maintain the status quo.

A Paradigm for Change

Kurt Lewin and his group of social scientists have studied factors facilitating or inhibiting change, and they offer the following:

1. Resistance to change:
   —increases in proportion to the degree to which it is perceived as a threat,
   —increases in response to direct pressure for change,
   —decreases when it is perceived as being favored by trusted others, those whose judgment is respected, and people of like mind,
   —decreases when those involved are able to foresee how they may establish a new equilibrium as good as or better than the old.
2. Resistance to change based on fear of the new circumstance is decreased when the individual has the opportunity to experience the new situation under conditions of minimal threat.
3. Commitment to change increases if the individual is a participant in decision making. [Lewin 1947]

Lewin offers a paradigm to assess change and plan strategies for change; this paradigm is called force-field analysis. The paradigm consists of an equilibrium resulting from the action of opposing forces that are equal in strength to one another. Lewin suggests that any equilibrium maintained by opposing forces would show a continuous fluctuation around a level within a fairly restricted range; that is, a quasi-stationary equilibrium. For this equilibrium to continue, any minor increase in one set of forces should be followed by a corresponding, compensatory increase in the opposing set of forces.

Here's an example: A nurse has a longing for independence and control and wants to start her own business; she has not yet decided to go into her own business. This nurse falls somewhere along the continuum between deciding to start a business and deciding not to start a business. If all the forces acting on her were in the direction of starting a business, she would move toward that end of the continuum and start her own business. If all the forces acting on her were opposed to starting her own business, she would decide not to do so. (See Figure 12-2.)

Driving forces, in this example, are all those factors that move an individual in the direction of the decision of going into business; restraining forces are all those factors that move an individual away from going into business. There could be any number of possible driving forces, among which might be:

1. Desire for independence, control, autonomy
2. Opinion and encouragement of friends
3. Ability in leadership, problem-solving
4. Desire for creative effort

Included in the restraining forces might be:

1. Expense of starting a business, and lack of money
2. Fear of failure
3. Lack of experience and knowledge of the business world
4. Unresolved dependency needs (i.e., wanting to be taken care of, or to be dependent)

For the situation to remain the same, each increase in driving forces would have to be met by an increase in restraining forces. To change the situation—that is, the level of the equilibrium—Lewin suggests modification of forces in three ways:

1. Increasing the driving forces by strengthening existing ones or adding new factors
2. Reducing or removing restraining forces
3. Letting a restraining force become a driving force

The most effective way to change the equilibrium is to modify in the first and second way simultaneously; that is, to find a way to increase driving forces and reduce restraining forces at the same time. The nurse deciding to go into business could increase the driving forces by taking college courses in business or management, or by enrolling in a master's in business administration program. She could also explore the possibilities of taking a job in a health care oriented business that would offer opportunities to learn management or

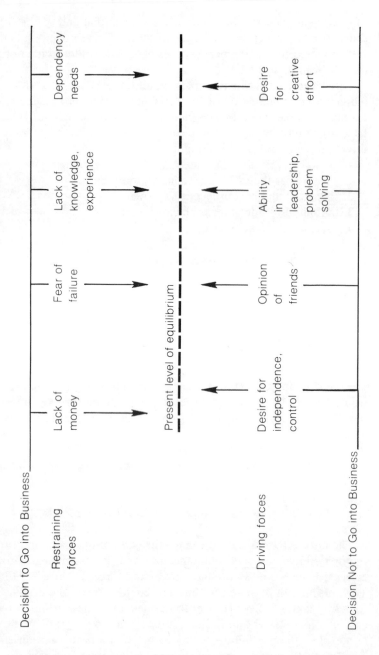

Figure 12-2   Quasi-stationary equilibrium of nurse undecided about going into her own business.

business skills. Any of these choices would also have an effect on the restraining forces of lack of knowledge and experience in the business world. In addition, she could associate with a group of women in business and work toward increasing her friends and business contacts. This aspect is considered in the discussion of networking in Chapter 11.

One could let restraining forces become driving forces in these ways:

1. Making a financial assessment with the help of an adviser from the Small Business Administration, and applying for a loan to initiate a small business

2. Applying for a grant or loan to get a master's or PhD in a specific content area in which the government identifies a need for more nurses, and which the nurse identifies as helpful to her future business plans

3. Working with a therapist or mental health counselor to increase awareness of dependency needs and to explore alternatives to learn to nurture and take care of oneself in an independent way

Force-field analysis is a helpful paradigm to use in becoming aware of resistance to change and in developing strategies to work with resistance. Theoretically, any of the forces in the field are subject to change; some are easier to change than others. The most efficient and effective tactic is to work on the restraining forces that can be changed with the least effort.

In using a force-field analysis as part of planning change, it is important to assess the forces that are latent in the situation, such as those that will become manifest as the level of equilibrium moves toward the goal. In the example, feelings of fear of failure may decrease as small successes are experienced; new business contacts may open doors to increased experiences or opportunity. Hope increases as experience and knowledge of nurses in business increase.

Many other forces affect the situation; in the example given, national health trends, political decisions about financial aid to small business or to women, education grants, accessibility of university classes, financial advice, and psychotherapy are some of the forces to assess.

The process of force-field analysis should be carried out repeatedly during the change process; each change in the situation changes the balance and calls for a new analysis until the desired goal is reached.

The Role of Awareness in Change

Becoming aware of what we are doing is the first step of change.
We then have choices: for example, shall I continue doing the same
thing, or shall I do something else? Until I am aware of that which I
do, I am probably going to continue in the same way. With
awareness comes choice. The following are ways to increase
awareness of self:

- Pay attention to your own behavior: "What is it that I do?"
- Pay attention to your feelings
- Write in a journal or diary
- Make lists of: I want . . .
                   I don't want . . .
                   I like . . .
                   I don't like . . .
                   My best vacation was . . .
                   My worst vacation was . . .
- Meditate
- Do yoga exercises
- Give yourself time to daydream, to wonder
- Learn relaxation techniques
- Work with biofeedback
- Keep a dream journal
- Ask friends, family, co-workers for feedback on how they experience you
- Participate in body movement or dance
- Participate in art, music, sculpting, or drama
- Join a women's support group
- Participate in individual or group psychotherapy
- Speak thoughts and ideas into a tape recorder; keep and play later to pick up patterns
- Learn to use imagery to explore self
- Do force-field analysis in decision making
- Read philosophy, psychology, and other literature that evokes curiosity and wonder about the human condition
- Use I-language; "I-language involves revelations of the speaker's feelings as well as reactions to the person spoken with. Feelings include emotional states, psychosomatic manifestations, skin sensations, postural ones, etc." (Marcus 1979, p. 25).

Change starts as we become aware and let ourselves observe and know ourselves. Do you remember, "This is the watchbird, watching YOU"? This was a series of cartoons in a magazine when I was growing up. As I remember, the watchbird was judgmental and moralistic; the watchbird watched in dichotomies of good and bad, right and wrong. Many of us watch ourselves in the same way. But this method of watching self is less than helpful, for we often tend to be supercritical and negative, hard on ourselves, and miss positive aspects. Awareness of self without judgment is the key to change.

Factors that inhibit awareness include these:

- Judgment
- Pride
- Fear
- Threat
- Negativity
- Lack of focus
- Having to be right, good, perfect
- Embarrassment
- Shame
- Guilt
- Rigidity
- Anger

If we can suspend judgment and reduce the other factors that inhibit awareness, it is possible to develop an observer self; the observer self can be like a researcher and collect data. Sometimes the observer self observes behaviors we don't want to own or know. If we are able to observe the behavior and know we don't want to know about that part of ourselves, a change has already taken place. An example might be the nurse who wants to start her own business and discovers that she procrastinates and has trouble setting her own deadlines to get work done. If she does not become an observer, she might never become aware of her procrastination and trouble with setting deadlines. If she lets herself become aware, she then has choices; she can continue in the same way or try an alternative way.

Here is another paradox: when I let myself know what I am doing to keep from changing, I have already begun to change by making the change of letting myself know!

"At its best, awareness is a continuous means for keeping up to date with one's self. It is an ongoing process . . . like an underground stream, ready to be tapped into when needed, a refreshing and revitalizing experience" (Polster and Polster 1974, p. 213). Awareness is a helpful tool; certainly, there are times when we are unaware and spontaneous, letting go of our observer and letting ourselves just be.

Strategies for Risk Taking

We use our imaginations to scare ourselves; "What if . . . ?" "They won't like it." "I'll make a fool of myself." Most of us are very good at scaring ourselves. Let yourself be open to the idea that the better you are at scaring yourself, the better you will be at using your imagination to grow and change.

Alternatives to Scaring Yourself

Imagination is energy that can be used to move toward a desired goal; instead of using your imagination to scare yourself, imagine yourself doing the new behavior beautifully and with ease. This positive image will then pull you toward what you want. More and more I am convinced that we must imagine a new behavior before we can do it; an active imagination gives the nervous system a trial run at the desired behavior, an imaginary practice.

In my practice as a mental health counselor, my clients often say, "I'm scared and uncomfortable; I can't do it," as if being scared and taking a new action were mutually exclusive. To go with the risk, it is necessary to say, "I'm scared and uncomfortable and I want to explore this risky place and see what is really there for me in the here and now." Curiosity is a strength that can lead to change.

Situations that we have anticipated with fear often turn out to be intriguing; the fear is a response from childhood or an earlier time when we lacked experience or skill. Each of us has an unexplored part of our personality, someone we would like to be or something we would like to do that we are reluctant to let ourselves explore. The Jungians speak of the disowned part, the dark side. This unexplored part might be our softness, our ability to write, dance, create, our vulnerability, our power, and so on. We inhibit and scare ourselves and so the part remains unexplored.

If you find that you are inhibiting yourself from exploring a part of yourself or a situation that seems risky, here are some positive ways to disinhibit yourself:

- Laughter
- Relaxation exercises
- Diaphragmatic breathing
- Dancing the new behavior
- Role playing with a friend
- Singing the new behavior
- Saying it out loud to a trusted friend
- Being childlike: swing on swings, make sand castles
- Using imagery to explore self, practice new behaviors, daydream
- Remembering past successes; telling them to a friend
- Brainstorming: look at plans and ideas without judgment; just write them on paper or say them into a tape recorder quickly. Don't edit or prejudge. Let yourself imagine that the words are waiting to tumble out and that you just need to give them the opportunity to be free.
- Finding someone who is doing the risky behavior: spend time with them; observe and learn.

The risk taker can learn to "hedge the risk," or protect herself by studying the situation and laying the groundwork for change. An example is using a checklist to survey the market if you want to go into business:

What Services/Products Will You Provide?
- Will they be the same as others now available?
- How will yours differ?
- What is your rationale for choosing them?
- Will you sell whatever people will buy?
- Will these services generate income for you?
- Will you start out with one service/product or several?
- What are your qualifications to provide the service, produce the product? (See Neal 1981.)

Other ways to hedge the risk of going into business include:

- Getting information
- Learning skills, theory, and process
- Being versatile and cultivating self-development in several different related areas
- Having reliable job skills to fall back on in rough times

Using Personal Power

"There is in every organism, at whatever level, an underlying flow of movement toward constructive fulfillment of its inherent possibilities . . . the term that has most often been used for this is the actualizing tendency" (Rogers 1977, p. 7). The growing edge is the place where actualizing takes place; in that growing edge, the known and the unknown meet. This place of risk is the transition and connection to the next level of experience. Going with the risk leads to growth; saying "yes" to risk connects the past, present, and future in a positive way. As we come to the growing edge, we are at a place of potential personal power, the unknown place, the place where the "wild things" exist. This is the place where Max, the child in Maurice Sendak's book *Where the Wild Things Are,* does his magic trick of taming the terrible wild things by saying, "Be still" and staring into their yellow eyes without blinking once. Max becomes powerful by confronting and focusing his awareness on the "wild things"; the wild things become tame, and later dance with Max. And so it is with each of us; we can get in touch with our personal power by letting ourselves risk awareness and confrontation in our own process.

Personal power, that inner strength that is expressed in vibrant, healthy, creative energy, is enhanced by:

- Being centered in your body
- Respecting self and others
- Trusting your own process
- Being aware of self, including strengths and weaknesses
- Having the ability to focus on your own feelings, hopes, ideals, attitudes
- Exploring your own reservations and unknown parts
- Making choices with responsibility
- Expressing feelings and ideas and getting feedback
- Staying in touch with the growing edge
- Making positive new tapes and playing them whenever you catch yourself in negative old tapes
- Going with the risk
- Saying "yes" to life
- Self-creation
- Self-actualization

Summary

The nurse who goes into business for herself enters into the process of risking and must develop strategies for adaptive coping with risk. I have discussed strategies for coping with risk, a paradigm for assessing change and developing strategies for change, the role of awareness in change, alternatives to scaring yourself, and enhancing personal power.

Going with the risk leads to the growing edge, with opportunity for creative learning and increased sense of personal power.

In closing, I would like to share that I had some reservations about writing this chapter in the first person and sharing my life experiences. As I discussed my feelings about this with a friend, he smiled and jotted down this poem:

risky business

me
   b
     e
      i
       n
        g
          here
sharing
       with
           strangers
              risky business

And so I conclude by sharing the risk with you, and inviting you to join me in going with the risk!

References

Capra, Fritjof. *The Tao of Physics.* New York: Bantam Books, 1977.

LeShan, Edna. *The Wonderful Crisis of Middle Age.* New York: David McKay, 1973.

Lewin, Kurt. "Group Decision and Social Change," in T. Newcomb, and E. Hartley (Eds.), *Readings in Social Psychology.* New York: Holt, Rinehart, and Winston, 1947.

Marcus, Eric. *Gestalt Therapy and Beyond.* Cupertino, California: Meta Publications, 1979.

May, Rollo. *The Courage to Create*. New York: Norton, 1975.

Neal, Margo C. "The Independent Provider: An Innovative Role," in Signe S. Cooper, and Margo C. Neal, (Eds.), *Perspectives on Continuing Education in Nursing*. Pacific Palisades, California: Nurseco, 1980.

Polster, Eving and Miriam. *Gestalt Therapy Integrated*. New York: Vintage Books, 1974.

Rogers, Carl. *On Personal Power*. New York: Delacorte, 1977.

Sendak, Maurice. *Where the Wild Things Are*. New York: Harper & Row, 1963.

Sheehy, Gail. *Passages*. New York: E.P. Dutton, 1976.

Webster's New Ideal Dictionary. Massachusetts: Merriam, 1973.

Bibliography

Klein, Donald. *Community Dynamics and Mental Health*. New York: Wiley, 1968.